THE FIBROMYALGIA HANDBOOK

THE
FIBROMYALGIA
HANDBOOK

HARRIS H. McILWAIN, M.D.
DEBRA FULGHUM BRUCE

AN OWL BOOK
HENRY HOLT AND COMPANY
NEW YORK

Henry Holt and Company, Inc.
Publishers since 1866
115 West 18th Street
New York, New York 10011

Henry Holt® is a registered
trademark of Henry Holt and Company, Inc.

Published in Canada by Fitzhenry & Whiteside Ltd.,
195 Allstate Parkway, Markham, Ontario L3R 4T8.

Library of Congress Cataloging-in-Publication Data
McIlwain, Harris H.
The fibromyalgia handbook / Harris H. McIlwain
and Debra Fulghum Bruce.
    p.   cm.
Includes bibliographical references and index.
1. Fibromyalgia—Handbooks, manuals, etc.
I. Bruce, Debra Fulghum.   II. Title.
RC927.3M36   1996   96-16846
616.7′4—dc20   CIP

ISBN 0-8050-4672-0

Henry Holt books are available for special
promotions and premiums. For details contact:
Director, Special Markets.

First Owl Book Edition—1996

Designed by Ann Gold

Printed in the United States of America
All first editions are printed on acid-free paper.∞

10 9 8 7 6 5

This book is not intended as a substitute for medical advice of physicians
and should be used only in conjunction with the advice of your personal doctor.
The reader should regularly consult a physician in matters relating to his or
her health and particularly with respect to any symptoms that may require
diagnosis or medical attention.

*To our parents, Cordelia McIlwain
and Roy and Jewel Fulghum,
for their love, devotion, and ongoing
encouragement to seek our dreams*

ACKNOWLEDGMENTS

The most important people in our lives, our families, deserve gold medals for patience and support as we prepared this manuscript. Without their help, this book would not be a reality. Our love goes to Linda, Laura, Kim, Michael, Ginah, and Daniel McIlwain; Bob, Rob, Brittnye, and Ashley Bruce; and Hugh Cruse.

We thank Sherry Buelow for the genuine feelings expressed so poignantly and hope that her lengthy experience with the disease can enable others to have hope.

To Lori Steinmeyer, M.S., R.D./L.D., we express gratitude. Your knowledge and experience with the nutritional healing of fibromyalgia patients, along with the belief that chronic illnesses can be managed through proper diet, adds timely insight to the book.

We are indebted to Laurence Smolley, M.D., pulmonologist with the Cleveland Clinic Florida. A sincere thank-you for the excellent wisdom about sleep disorders with fibromyalgia patients, along with your practical suggestions to enhance more restful sleep.

To Frank J. Novakoski, M.A., A.T.C., we greatly appreciate your knowledge of weight training with fibromyalgia patients along with your expertise in the field of exercise physiology.

Gratitude is expressed to Drs. Daniel and April Dodd. Your background in chiropractic with fibromyalgia patients enabled us to show a more comprehensive treatment mode for the reader.

To Judith Riven, our literary agent, our heartfelt thanks for believing in this topic for publication. Your devotion and persistence enabled us to secure the book with the right publisher.

Finally, to Cynthia Vartan, our editor, a special thank-you for your ongoing support and enthusiasm for this project. We are proud to be associated with Henry Holt and Company.

CONTENTS

THE FIBROMYALGIA HANDBOOK

INTRODUCTION:
YOU HAVEN'T GOT TIME
FOR THE PAIN

If you have been diagnosed with fibromyalgia, tension myalgia, fibrositis, or generalized rheumatism, no one needs to tell you of the almost daily muscle pain you live with, along with constant fatigue, sleeplessness, and low-grade depression. As a rheumatologist for more than twenty years, I have seen fibromyalgia take its toll on once healthy individuals, mostly women ages twenty to sixty. Not only does it strike during young and middle adult years, the busiest and most stressful time of one's life, but patients tell of the symptoms making them feel as if they are 100 years old. The good news is that *it does not have to be this way!* You can live actively with fibromyalgia, *if* you learn how to manage its symptoms with some specific lifestyle changes.

Years ago, it became apparent to doctors that patients who told of having muscle aches, fatigue, depression, headaches, and sleeplessness were harboring a distinct disease or syndrome (a collection of symptoms that make a disease). Yet the results from lab tests and X rays were always normal. Two decades ago, physicians sent these patients home with few answers, as we could only treat the symptoms.

Today we know differently. In the past five years there has been a plethora of research done on this mysterious syndrome we call "fibromyalgia." Now millions of people can understand that the disease is real; the symptoms are *not* imagined *nor* did they cause them; and treatment does work, if followed faithfully.

A View of Fibromyalgia

In this book, you will become knowledgeable about fibromyalgia and learn how to lessen the severity of the symptoms. Questions will be addressed, such as:

- Does being overweight make one more likely to get fibromyalgia?
- Is it inherited?
- Why is this considered a "female" disease?
- Does estrogen have anything to do with it?
- Is there a cure for this or will it continue to cause pain for my entire life?
- Should I push myself on days when the pain and fatigue seem unbearable?
- How do I know which medications will help me?
- How can my doctor know for sure that this is fibromyalgia?
- Will the disease run its course?
- Did I cause the disease from too much stress or poor nutrition?
- Does exercise hurt or help the painful symptoms?

While there are no cures for fibromyalgia, you can learn to control your specific symptoms as you manage the disease with the 7-Step Treatment Program. This plan has proved to be successful with thousands of my patients as they identify the symptoms of the disease, carefully seek a diagnosis, and learn to manage the disease in a reasonable way.

Let's look at some patients who have taken the steps

needed to control their fibromyalgia and are winning with this disease.

Chronic Fatigue and Muscle Pain

Linda was one patient who benefited greatly from the combination 7-Step Treatment Program outlined in this book. After her youngest child entered elementary school, this thirty-nine-year-old woman enrolled at the local university to work on her master's degree. Halfway through the quarter, Linda noticed a dramatic change in her health. "I've always needed eight hours of sleep," she said upon evaluation. "But for the past month, I have been sleeping eleven or twelve hours and still feel tired when I awaken."

This once active woman told of feeling so chronically fatigued that even walking to class from a nearby parking lot left her feeling weak. "Not only am I tired, but my muscles ache like I've been exercising too hard, yet I haven't worked out at all."

After seeing three physicians, including a sleep disorders specialist who ruled out any pulmonary problems, Linda came to our clinic. In the meantime, Linda continued to take courses while maintaining a family. But the added stress of going to school and studying took its toll, for she felt overwrought, as if her body was failing her.

Upon diagnosis, Linda began the 7-Step Treatment Program and her symptoms responded positively. Within three weeks, the symptoms lessened dramatically, and she finally found relief from the constant and nagging pain and fatigue.

Hot, Searing Leg Pain

Jean, a high school principal, told of being unable to walk one morning about five years ago. "I'll never forget that day for as long as I live. I had set my alarm early that morning because the accreditation team was coming to the school for our annual review.

"When I put my feet on the floor, my legs simply gave way. My left ankle had a hot, searing, and burning pain that went throughout the heel, arch, and toes. When I sat on my right hip, my thigh and leg hurt so badly, it was unbearable. There was a pinching feeling in my hip and I could hardly walk. All I could think of was that my career was over."

Jean's symptom of pain was so severe that it took several months to get this under control. However, as Linda also experienced, once Jean began the treatment plan in this book, she was able to live a more normal, active life again.

Achiness, Fatigue, and Depression

When Elizabeth, a forty-five-year-old attorney, got over a recent bout with the flu, she thought that the achiness that lingered was from being run-down. "I had this unending pain that made me so depressed. I even thought that death would be a welcome relief, because I hurt all over. The pain became so intense that I couldn't have sex with my husband without tears, yet he did not seem to understand. I couldn't even do light household chores without wanting to scream out in agony."

It took three months of doctor's appointments, until Elizabeth's symptoms were finally given a name—fibromyalgia. "How could doctors look me straight in the eye and say that the pain and fatigue were in my head? One doctor said that a cruise would make me feel less stressed. A cruise? I didn't need a cruise, I needed a diagnosis and form of treatment."

For Elizabeth, living with fibromyalgia has been an eye-opening experience. "It is hard to realize that healthy people can get this disease, but they can. I now understand that education is the key in controlling the symptoms."

Most important, the quality of life for Linda, Jean, and Elizabeth has greatly improved since starting the treatment plan. All three tell of now sleeping soundly, having more energy, and feeling less pressure since they took control of the debilitating symptoms.

From Patient to Person

What is the goal of living with this disease? You should strive to change the disease from something disabling to something manageable. With the 7-Step Treatment Program, you can learn to treat each symptom in a positive manner, doing the activities you enjoy in reasonable comfort without being overly medicated or feeling debilitating pain and stiffness.

You deserve to know that the high anxiety that accompanies fibromyalgia can make you feel broken, especially when you haven't got time for the pain, fatigue, and immobility. However, in the midst of the brokenness that you feel, I know that you can become a *whole person* again as you learn to conquer this disease instead of conceding to it.

Now let's get started.

1

WHAT IS FIBROMYALGIA?

We all get tired. And who doesn't feel sore, achy, and stiff, especially after a weekend of sports activities or heavy gardening? For those with fibromyalgia, these debilitating symptoms of pain and fatigue are severe and constant, lasting for months and years and causing poor quality of life for its millions of victims—damaging jobs, families, and personal lives.

Rebecca came to our clinic because of widespread pain that she described as "stabbing and throbbing" from her shoulders and the back of her neck to her legs. This forty-seven-year-old woman worked full-time as a data processor, but in the past few months she had been unable to sit at the computer for any length of time due to the pain.

"I wake up every day with stabbing pain and think that maybe it will go away," she said. "When I get to work and sit at the computer, the pain worsens and often feels piercing, like a knife is in my muscle. I feel tired all the time and can't cook dinner for my family. If anyone touches me, I cringe because of the tenderness. Because of the exhaustion, I'm in bed by 7:30 P.M. each night, yet I never feel rested. What is wrong with me?"

After a careful examination and evaluation of the symptoms, this middle-aged woman was diagnosed with fibromyalgia. Coined in 1976, the term *fibromyalgia* describes the basic symptoms of constant muscle pain, tenderness, fatigue, and tender points. As Rebecca experienced, fibromyalgia causes widespread pain—in the back, neck, arms, and legs—with many tender or trigger points that are very painful when touched.

Fibromyalgia—with its deep muscle pain, disturbed sleep, and feelings of depression—affects more than 10 million Americans, with 90 percent or more being women aged forty to fifty or older. Sophisticated research has shown that the disease can start in childhood or teenage years, especially with girls, and gradually worsens with age. Some recent studies show that because of the common symptoms, the disease may be vastly underdiagnosed in older adults, who often accept the unexplained pain in their bodies as another sign of aging. It is important to know up front that fibromyalgia is *not* a sign of aging!

Patients tell of going from doctor to doctor with symptoms of fatigue, which are present even on arising. They may have specific *tender points* on the body that hurt to the touch, or they may have pain all over. Forty-one-year-old Janis told of hurting everywhere on her body; even sitting in a straight-back chair brought tears to her eyes. Sarah, a young mother of two, felt throbbing pain all over her body as well as disturbances in deep-level, restful sleep, accompanied by sadness or depression. Mike felt a piercing pain in his neck and shoulders, accompanied by sluggishness, that came on suddenly after a car accident. While these patients had different manifestations of pain and fatigue, the symptoms were all the result of fibromyalgia.

A Common but Misunderstood Disease

Even though this has been a commonly misdiagnosed and misunderstood syndrome, fibromyalgia is the most common arthritis-related disease next to osteoarthritis. The consensus document on fibromyalgia from the Second World Conference on Myofascial Pain and Fibromyalgia in 1992 reported that fibromyalgia may be the most common cause of widespread musculoskeletal pain.

Fibromyalgia was first described in medical documents more than 150 years ago, yet even as recent as ten years ago, this disease was rarely discussed in the medical community. Those who don't understand it may not recognize that it exists. One middle-aged woman recently brought her entire family into our clinic to talk about the disease. "Because I look healthy, they think I overexaggerate my symptoms," she explained. "Please tell them that I'm not making this up."

One must wonder how treatment can begin if the problem is not recognized. For most people, it is common for the symptoms to drag on for months or years before a proper diagnosis is made. In fact, for most patients, the average amount of time to pass before diagnosis is made is *4 to 5 years.* Imagine living half a decade with debilitating symptoms and being told by family, friends, and your physician that the pain and fatigue are probably in your head!

Thousands of patients each year tell of going from doctor to doctor with symptoms of crippling fatigue and constant muscle and joint pain all over their body. "Before I was diagnosed with fibromyalgia, I was told by two doctors that nothing was wrong with me," Vicky said, "and another suggested that my pain was psychological."

While more and more people are receiving the proper diagnosis of fibromyalgia from physicians who understand this rheumatic type disease, there are estimates that thousands of people are still living with undiagnosed and untreated symptoms. If you have been diagnosed with fibromyalgia or if you have the described symptoms and believe that this might be the problem, you have probably heard one or more of the following statements from friends and family members:

"It's all in your head."
"If you would relax more, you could sleep at night."
"Maybe you're too focused on yourself; get out and get busy."
"If you would exercise more, you wouldn't feel that muscle pain."
"Get a job. It will make you feel less depressed."
"You look healthy to me. Maybe you just want sympathy."
"You just don't want to feel good. Why do you always crave attention?"
"Slow down. Your life is so busy, it is making you crazy."
"Your life is wonderful, so don't be depressed."
"If the doctor says it's in your head, it must be true."
"If the lab tests do not show anything, you aren't sick."
"You act like this is the end of the world; lighten up."

After suffering with endless pain and chronic fatigue day after day, month after month, you may even begin to believe that you are fabricating the symptoms or that the problem really is in your mind. But this disease is very real.

Lydia, a forty-two-year-old lab technician and mother of two, was faced with early retirement due to the fatigue and even had to take catnaps throughout her workday to keep going. Lydia told of feeling widespread aching and stabbing pain in her muscles and joints, which greatly affected her ability to work and care for her family. She lived with these symptoms for four years and was evaluated by six doctors but did not receive a successful diagnosis.

When she came to our clinic, she felt tired, achy, and mildly depressed. But more important, Lydia was angry that no one could tell her what was happening to her body. "I guess because my symptoms and feelings come and go, the doctors thought that I was overworked or depressed," she said. "The antidepressant one doctor prescribed helped my sleep, but I still didn't feel rested in the morning, and I continued to hurt all over."

Darlene came to our clinic complaining of searing pain in her back, neck, and chest, along with throbbing headaches that occurred almost daily. This forty-five-year-old legal secretary and single mother of three had very specific *tender points* on the body that were painful to touch, along with regular disturbances in deep-level or restful sleep at night. Her main concern was the stiffness throughout her body on arising in the morning. "I have to work, but after walking up the stairs to my office, the pain is unbearable," she said.

Darlene's excruciating pain was worsened by any stress, a symptom which is quite common. She said that when the disease was active, her concentration at work was gravely affected, and she felt more irritable, even depressed. Another patient, forty-year-old Nina, had deep muscle pain in the abdomen along with dramatic changes in her bowel habits, ranging from constipation to diarrhea.

Darlene and Nina had frequency in urination with a sensation of an immediate urge to urinate; and both women complained of painful menstrual cramps, which are quite common in women with fibromyalgia. Nina had a pale discoloration of the fingers on cold exposure, such as holding a cold glass or putting the hand in the refrigerator.

Sick or Old?

Peter, a middle-aged gentleman, came to see me about his symptoms, which had been ongoing for several months. He seemed a bit nervous during our conversation, then admitted that on the day of his evaluation, he was symptom-free. "I don't understand it," Peter said. "The past few days, I didn't ache at all, and last night I slept for the first time without tossing and turning."

Peter's case is not unusual. In fibromyalgia, the symptoms may come and go; therefore, it may be difficult to get proper diagnosis. If the physician does not understand the complexity of the disease, a patient may be sent away without any help or hope for treatment. In fact, studies show that *thousands* of patients each year tell of going from doctor to doctor with constant pain all over their body along with feelings of fatigue. Many are told that there is nothing wrong or that the problem is psychological.

Today we know differently. We know that fibromyalgia is a complex disorder characterized by *chronic* (meaning three months or longer) widespread pain, decreased pain threshold or tender points, and incapacitating fatigue. Women are ten times more likely to get the disease than men. While there is no specific laboratory test or abnormal X ray finding for diagnosis, the symptoms of the disease can be successfully treated once a proper diagnosis is made.

The Causes of Fibromyalgia

A RESULT OF MENOPAUSE

"Since I went into menopause, my symptoms have quadrupled," Lois, a fifty-four-year-old retired teacher who was diagnosed three years ago, said. "I had to quit teaching kindergarten because the pain in my shoulders and neck kept me from keeping up with my kids, and I felt so tired each day."

Some researchers have suggested that the loss of the female hormone *estrogen*, which happens at menopause, may trigger this disease. Hosts of experiments are being done to see if loss of estrogen does, in fact, stimulate this disease; it is true that fibromyalgia occurs more commonly between the ages of forty to fifty-five, or around the time of menopause.

DUE TO AGING

"Maybe fibromyalgia is similar to aging," Nancy surmised. "All these symptoms came on at midlife, and I have heard that all things fall apart after age forty."

The truth is that even though the disease occurs more frequently after the age of forty, there is no specific evidence that fibromyalgia is a problem of aging. It is also well known to occur in teenagers and gradually worsen over time. It does not continue to increase in much older people (seventy to eighty years old).

CONNECTED TO SEROTONIN OR MAGNESIUM DEFICIENCY

Clearly, some research indicates that other possible causes could be a deficiency of one of the body's chemicals, *serotonin,* or its precursor, *tryptophan,* or even magnesium. While there is still some controversy, some researchers have shown that abnormal levels of serotonin and other substances might explain the increase in pain that patients feel. These findings might also explain the sleep problems associated with this disease.

AFTER THE FLU OR AS A RESULT OF LYME DISEASE

Fibromyalgia often occurs following an injury, even one that may be mild, or after a bout with the flu. Some patients diagnosed with Lyme disease, which can cause muscle and joint pain, along with other problems, and is spread through the bite of a tick, were found to have fibromyalgia as their main problem. No specific evidence was found that Lyme disease caused fibromyalgia in those patients.

POOR PHYSICAL CONDITIONING OR AS A RESULT OF DEPRESSION

Some studies support the theory that people who are unfit are more likely to get fibromyalgia. Speculation is that stress and poor physical conditioning may both be major factors in the cause of the disease.

Other studies have shown that because fibromyalgia is accompanied by low-grade depression, there may be a link between these two illnesses. Some researchers feel that depression leads to changes in the chemistry of the brain or that abnormalities of the sympathetic nervous system result in the release of substances that cause more sensitivity to pain, resulting in fibromyalgia.

LINKED TO STRESS OR TRAUMA TO NERVOUS SYSTEM

Mounting evidence indicates that fibromyalgia is linked to stress or emotional illness. On the other hand, some studies show that psychological stress in the patient is often high *before* the disease begins. Although it is not known why, researchers are finding that fibromyalgia may be caused by biochemical changes in the body, for example, accidents, injuries, or illnesses. Other studies reveal that the disease may result from sudden trauma to the central nervous system.

UNKNOWN CAUSES

While there are many theories on what causes fibromyalgia, the truth remains unknown. For many years doctors thought that the disease was caused by a disorder of the muscles or that it was a psychological problem. Some researchers believe that this mysterious syndrome has a genetic disposition, as it can run in families. The most recent research suggests that the muscles themselves are not the source of the pain, but rather that the pain is a response to changes in the brain. All of these explanations remain unproven, but research is continuing.

No single theory seems to explain all of the problems in fibromyalgia. Whatever the cause, the vicious cycle of pain and disturbed sleep leads to less activity, greater depression, and more pain. This pain cycle can incapacitate the sufferer for months and possibly years unless the proper treatment is administered to control the symptoms. While there is no cure, the symptoms *can* be successfully treated.

Fibromyalgia and Other Illnesses

If what current research indicates is true, other factors play a role in increasing or lessening fibromyalgia's symptoms. We know that when other illnesses or diseases are present, symptoms can greatly accelerate, causing more pain, fatigue, and anxiety or depression. The disease can worsen during times of great stress or after exercise. Conversely, the chronic pain can subside during less stressful times. Beverly, age thirty-seven, told of living with chronic pain for months. Then, during a two-week cruise to the Caribbean with her husband, she became almost pain-free.

"After a few days into the cruise, I started sleeping through the night without awakening, and I was able to sightsee without resting periodically for the muscle pain. I thought I was healed, except that it was short-lived.

"Almost one month after my vacation, the pain started again, and it was worse than ever. Somehow, I know that lessening my stress helped me stay symptom-free."

FIBROMYALGIA CLASSIFICATIONS
1. Fibromyalgia without any other underlying disease, such as osteoarthritis or other types of arthritis.
2. Fibromyalgia along with another disease, such as osteoarthritis, rheumatoid arthritis, or systemic lupus erythematosus (SLE).

The Feelings of Fibromyalgia

Because fibromyalgia can cause signs and feelings similar to osteoarthritis, bursitis, and tendinitis, some specialists include it in the group of arthritis and related disorders. But unlike the bursitis or tendinitis, which is usually localized to a single area, the feelings of pain and stiffness associated with fibromyalgia are widespread. In fact, if there are not many areas involved, then it does not fit the typical picture of fibromyalgia. If a joint is warm or swollen or does not move properly, then there is probably another problem present, such as another form of arthritis or an injury.

For some patients, fibromyalgia's symptoms are not always chronic—the pain comes and goes. Unlike some severe forms of arthritis that cause crippling, most fibromyalgia patients are able to get through the day, though they constantly feel tired and achy.

COMMON SYMPTOMS OF FIBROMYALGIA
Pain
Fatigue
Morning stiffness
Trigger points
Sleep problems
Anxiety
Difficulty in concentration
Depression
Swelling, numbness, and tingling in hands, arms, feet,
    and legs
Headaches
Irritable bowel syndrome
Urinary symptoms
Painful menstrual cramps
Discoloration of hands and feet (Raynaud's phenomenon)

Restless legs syndrome
Dryness in mouth, nose, and eyes

PAIN: THE MOST COMMON SYMPTOM

Pain plays a significant role in the diagnosis of fibromyalgia and is usually the major complaint that signals a visit to the doctor. This widespread pain is characteristic of more than 97 percent of patients. Unlike the pain of osteoarthritis, bursitis, or tendinitis, which is usually relegated to a specific joint or area, this pain can be felt over the entire body and is deep, sharp, dull, throbbing, or aching. There may also be accompanying pain in the joints, such as the shoulders, hips, back, and neck. Joint pain can also come from the hands, wrists, elbows, ankles, and feet. However, even more common is pain felt in the muscles, tendons, and ligaments around the joints.

Peggy was diagnosed strictly from the pain she was experiencing. "I live day and night with a sharp, throbbing pain in the muscles in my neck and shoulders, yet I have not experienced the fatigue that usually accompanies this. The pain became especially intense after exercise or housework, especially when I do such chores as sweeping, mopping, vacuuming, or washing windows. The pain becomes so unbearable that even over-the-counter pain medications do not touch it."

Other patients who tell of feeling pain in the back, neck, and head complain also of frequent headaches. Many times these pains are from the muscles and other soft tissues around the back and neck, not from fibromyalgia.

I often see patients who have had a back injury, such as a ruptured disc in the lower part of the spine (lumbar spine). These patients have had surgery on the lower back or neck for treatment of the injury. However, for unknown reasons many of these patients develop symptoms of fibromyalgia after a back injury, which may result in forced bed rest, along with loss of activity.

RELENTLESS FATIGUE IS CRIPPLING

Next to pain and the tender trigger points, fatigue is a major complaint. We *all* know what it feels like to be tired. However, because we are each different, we may have dissimilar ideas of the meaning of *fatigue.* What is fatigue to you may not be the same for me or someone else. Fatigue in fibromyalgia refers to a lingering tiredness that is constant and limiting. For example, patients complain of being tired even when they should feel rested and have had enough sleep. Some patients admit to feeling sleepy, but much more common is a feeling of exhaustion without feeling drowsy. Some compare it to having the flu or to the feeling after working very long hours and missing a lot of sleep.

Just as the cause of fibromyalgia is not known, the exact cause of the fatigue is not known. Sleep disturbances, common in the large majority of patients, may help create a constant state of fatigue. In fact, hosts of experiments have shown that many of fibromyalgia's symptoms can actually be created in otherwise healthy people if their sleep is disturbed. Fatigue is so bothersome in many patients that they often say, "Please get rid of the fatigue, and I'll put up with the pain."

THE FATIGUE OF FIBROMYALGIA

Fatigued on arising in the morning
Fatigued after mild activity, such as grocery shopping or cooking dinner
Too fatigued to start a project, such as folding clothes or ironing
Too fatigued to exercise
Even more fatigued after exercise
Too fatigued for sex
Too fatigued to function adequately at work

MORNING STIFFNESS AFFECTS MOST PATIENTS

More than 75 percent of fibromyalgia patients feel stiffness in the morning on arising. This stiffness creates a feeling of the need to loosen up after getting out of bed before usual activities can begin, and the stiffness is extensive, going throughout the muscles and joints of the back, arms, and legs. In some patients, the morning stiffness may last only a few minutes, but it is usually very noticeable for more than fifteen or twenty minutes each day. Other patients report that the stiffness lasts for hours or even seems to be present all day. Most people feel stiff when they wake up, but this type of stiffness is very different than minor aching. In fact, this is the same feeling of stiffness in the morning that happens in many types of arthritis, especially rheumatoid arthritis.

TRIGGER POINTS

Many influences are at work in fibromyalgia. Patients like Peggy feel sharp, throbbing muscle pain. But accompanying this deep muscle soreness are painful *trigger points,* or localized areas of tenderness around joints (not joints themselves), that hurt when pressed with a finger. These are often not deep areas of pain, but rather superficial areas seemingly under the surface of the skin, such as over the elbow or shoulder.

The cause of these trigger points is not known. Even though it would seem that these areas should be inflamed, no particular signs of inflammation have been found by researchers when the tissues are examined. The locations of the trigger points are not random; they are in predictable places on the body (see page 32).

DEPRESSION INTERFERES WITH ACTIVITIES

Depression is a key symptom with most patients. In fact, anxiety and depression severe enough to interfere with daily activities occur in fifty percent or more of fibromyalgia patients. Stress from the constant pain and fatigue can cause anxiety. The chronic pain can result in less activity, leading the patient to become more withdrawn, which can lead to depression.

No matter which case is eventually found to be correct, anxiety and depression can greatly interfere with a patient's activities at work and at home. The symptoms can be successfully treated with a combination of medication and therapy, so it is important to discuss these feelings openly with your doctor.

Patients also tell of having great difficulty concentrating on their work, along with intermittently impaired short-term memory.

SWELLING AND TINGLING HANDS CAN BE A PROBLEM

While the cause is not known, many patients have a feeling of swelling in the hands, arms, feet, or legs. The feeling may be especially bothersome upon arising, especially in combination with morning stiffness, yet does not appear to limit activity.

Numbness or tingling sensations in the hands, arms, or legs are also reported by more than half of all fibromyalgia patients. The medical term for these feelings is *paresthesia*. The sensations happen irregularly and usually last a few minutes, though they can be constant. While these sensations may be bothersome, they are not severely limiting.

CHRONIC HEADACHES ARE PART OF THE DISEASE

More than half of all fibromyalgia patients suffer from chronic headaches. They are often caused by tightness in and contraction of the muscles of the neck and are called *tension-type headaches* or *muscle-contraction headaches*. They may also be caused by tenderness from trigger points over the back of the head and the neck. It is important to remember that headaches can be caused by other medical problems, which should be properly diagnosed and treated by your doctor.

IRRITABLE BOWEL SYNDROME AFFECTS SUFFERERS
Irritable bowel syndrome (IBS) is a condition characterized by abdominal cramps and pain, along with periods of diarrhea alternating with bouts of constipation. About one-third of fibromyalgia patients suffer from IBS. Complaints can include excessive gas and bloating along with the irritable bowel syndrome.

URINARY FREQUENCY CAN OCCUR
A feeling of the urge to urinate, which is a condition called *urinary frequency,* painful urination, and incontinence have been found in about 25 percent of fibromyalgia patients. Since these problems can also be caused by other bladder and kidney diseases, it is important to check with your doctor to be sure no other specific problems are present.

PAINFUL MENSTRUAL CRAMPS AFFECT FEMALE PATIENTS
Unusually painful menstrual cramps are found in 30 to 40 percent of women with fibromyalgia. There are specific problems that can cause menstrual cramps, so be sure to check with your doctor to be sure no other treatment is needed.

DISCOLORATION OF EXTREMITIES
Some patients notice that their fingers or, though less commonly, their toes become pale, cold, or turn blue when exposed to cold—even such a small exposure as holding a cold glass. The pale or blue changes may last for a few minutes and can be accompanied by pain. When the hands or feet are warmed, they return to normal.

This problem is called *Raynaud's phenomenon.* It can happen in otherwise normal persons and is also a characteristic of other medical problems, such as other types of arthritis. Again, your doctor can be sure no other medical problems are present. Sometimes, medications are needed to control this symptom.

RESTLESS LEGS SYNDROME

Restless legs syndrome is a condition many fibromyalgia sufferers complain of. This is characterized by discomfort of the legs, especially below the knee, and is especially bothersome at night. The feeling can be painful and is most commonly described as the need to move the legs to try to make them comfortable. Restless legs syndrome often interrupts sleep as the sufferer tries to find the most comfortable position for rest. As with other symptoms, restless legs syndrome can be found with other medical problems and has no good treatment.

DRYNESS IS A CONCERN

Dryness of the mouth, nose, or eyes can happen in otherwise normal persons but more than 25 percent of fibromyalgia patients have this symptom. Dryness occurs when glands do not produce the normal amounts or quality of tears to lubricate the eyes or saliva to lubricate the mouth. This problem is commonly associated with rheumatoid and other types of arthritis and is called *Sjögren's syndrome*. There is no single known cause.

Although dryness is mainly uncomfortable, the loss of normal lubrication for the eyes can increase the risk of infection. The loss of normal saliva and lubrication in the mouth increases the chance of tooth decay. See your ophthalmologist and/or dentist for treatment.

Factors That Worsen Symptoms

In many studies, patients report that weather changes greatly affect musculoskeletal symptoms. In fact, those with the highest weather sensitivity tend to have more functional impairment and psychological distress.

FACTORS THAT CAN WORSEN FIBROMYALGIA SYMPTOMS
Fatigue
Changes in weather (cold or humidity)
Periods of emotional stress
Physical exhaustion
Lack of sleep or restless sleep
Sedentary lifestyle
Anxiety and depression

Fibromyalgia with Other Diseases

Fibromyalgia can occur alone or it can occur with one of the other 100 types of arthritis. For example, you may have osteoarthritis in the knee from an old football injury; yet you can have fibromyalgia in addition to this. Not only would you be faced with pain and stiffness in your knee, but the fibromyalgia would cause pain in the neck, back, shoulders, arms, legs, and hips; widespread stiffness accompanied by fatigue; depression; and headache.

It is also fairly common to see fibromyalgia in patients with rheumatoid arthritis. In fact, studies show that more than 20 percent of persons with rheumatoid arthritis also have fibromyalgia. Rheumatoid arthritis causes chronic pain and swelling in the joints of the hands, wrists, elbows, shoulders, knees, ankles, feet, and other joints. Other symptoms include morning stiffness and fatigue. While some patients definitely have rheumatoid arthritis, they also have all of the typical findings of fibromyalgia. Other forms of arthritis commonly occur along with fibromyalgia, including osteoarthritis, systemic lupus erythematosus (SLE or lupus), psoriatic arthritis, or polymyalgia rheumatica. Having one type of arthritis does not prevent you from also developing fibromyalgia!

The disease can also happen in patients who have chronic back pain, injuries to the back or neck, or a ruptured lumbar or cervical disc, as well as internal organ diseases.

Fibromyalgia Increases Depression

As sufferers live with the symptoms of fibromyalgia, they can become more and more focused on their pain and sadness, which is very real. The many appointments with health care providers to try to find relief, combined with the cost of these attempts, add to the patient's frustration.

As time goes on, patients have trouble keeping a job because of their many absences. As income declines, there can be more financial stresses to be dealt with by the sufferer and family. These stresses, along with the constant fatigue, pain, and low-grade depression, can cause severe relationship problems in the family.

The longer the situation lasts, the more likely a patient will see signs of stress, including:

Constant tiredness
Difficulty concentrating
Increasing irritability
Withdrawal from other activities (especially enjoyable ones)
Change in appetite
Depression

Each of us shows stress in different ways. If you have been diagnosed with fibromyalgia or think that you may have this disease, it is important to try to understand the ways in which you show stress that accompanies the disease. Then you can begin steps to control the stress (see chapters 5 and 6).

The Cost of Fibromyalgia

In addition to the human cost in suffering to the patient and family, the expenses associated with this disease can be devastating. Health care and medication costs can run to many thousands of dollars, not including the costs of specialized tests, counseling, or hospitalization.

After an extended course of treatment with little control of pain and more loss of activity, patients may be referred to a pain clinic. An inpatient pain clinic with a four-to-six-week treatment can be helpful, but this alone may cost $20,000 or more.

The good news is that large savings in health care costs are possible if the symptoms can be controlled. And the improvement in human costs could affect millions of people.

Take a Proactive Approach to Healing

The fact is, the outlook for people with fibromyalgia is remarkably better than ever before. Ongoing research and scientific trials are providing new information on the disease and how to treat the symptoms successfully. However, the first step in controlling these symptoms is understanding all you can about the disease, including the recommended modes of treatment and seeking a proper diagnosis, which is explained in chapter 2. Most patients feel a noticeable decrease in pain and fatigue and an increase in mobility and energy within a few months of starting treatment. This is exactly what happened to Helen, who has lived with this mysterious disease for two years.

This young attorney told of having throbbing muscle pain when she was in law school. "I was so stressed all the time from trying to compete in my class that I just assumed that the pain and tiredness I felt were caused by this," she told me.

"But when I left law school and joined a large practice in town, I continued to have the same symptoms."

Helen lived with undiagnosed fibromyalgia and quietly suffered its life-stealing symptoms—working her school schedule around daily nap periods and avoiding heavy activity or sports for fear of more pain and fatigue. Today she is a different person. She has learned that while the symptoms still wax and wane, she can actively tackle these symptoms with lifestyle changes that make a difference in how she feels each day.

Everyone Is Different

Remember, each person is different. The more specific the diagnosis of arthritis and rheumatic diseases, the more specific the treatment can be. This book cannot replace a proper medical diagnosis. It was written to help you become more informed about fibromyalgia so that you can knowledgeably seek a professional diagnosis from your doctor and begin treatment.

MAKING
THE DIAGNOSIS

M aria came to see me after living with undiagnosed chronic muscle pain for more than six years. At age thirty-seven, this mother of three told of sleeping all morning after getting her children off to school, taking another late afternoon nap while her children watched TV, then going to bed before 8:00 P.M. When she wasn't sleeping, Maria described symptoms of chronic headache, irritable bowel syndrome, muscle tension, and tender areas that were painful when anyone touched her.

After ruling out other diseases, Maria was diagnosed with fibromyalgia. Even though she realized that there was no cure for this disease, Maria was relieved to know finally what was causing her daily discomfort and fatigue.

Another patient, Susan, had to face a great deal of anger that it had taken so long to make a diagnosis of her chronic sleep problems, depression, and muscle pain. "If I had known then what I know now, I wouldn't have spent more than two thousand dollars trying to find an answer. Half the battle of winning with this disease is knowing that you didn't make it up."

A Difficult Diagnosis

Many patients like Maria and Susan tell of traveling from doctor to doctor with fibromyalgia—without results—because there are no specific tests for the disease. It may be difficult to make an accurate diagnosis if you cannot see a scientific measurement, such as laboratory tests or X rays. This is why in years past, millions of cases were misdiagnosed as depression or chronic fatigue syndrome (CFS).

Normal Laboratory Tests

With today's high-tech medicine, we have become used to special testing, blood tests, or other expensive tests to arrive at a diagnosis. However, most laboratory tests are not very helpful by themselves in making the diagnosis of fibromyalgia. In fact, this is one medical problem in which talking with the patient may be the most important tool in arriving at the correct diagnosis. The reason for this is that the major points for diagnosis of fibromyalgia are discovered from the way that you feel. While a physical examination will show your doctor the painful trigger points, as discussed on page 36, even with trigger points, you must *tell* your doctor of the exact pain you feel in those areas.

Upon evaluation, your doctor will want to have a few basic laboratory tests taken to be sure no other serious medical problems are present. But these tests are limited in number and can be performed at your doctor's office or your local laboratory. They can usually all be done at one visit.

Specific Laboratory Tests Used

Some specific blood tests that your doctor may ask for include a complete blood count (CBC). This test measures hemoglobin levels and provides a count of red blood cells, white blood cells, and platelets. It is used to diagnose many common blood disorders, such as anemia, that can cause fatigue.

The chemistries in your blood will also be checked and will include blood tests that tell how the kidney and liver are functioning, cholesterol and other fats in the blood, calcium levels, and tests of other chemicals in the blood such as cholesterol "glucose," that can create problems similar to fibromyalgia, but which are treated differently. Thyroid tests will be done at the same time with blood tests to see if the thyroid is working properly.

Testing for Arthritis

If arthritis is a question, one test that may be included is the *erythrocyte sedimentation rate* (sed rate or ESR). This is an old test that measures the rate at which red blood cells settle out in a tube of unclotted blood; a higher than normal sed rate indicates inflammation. Patients with rheumatoid arthritis and other similar types of arthritis have abnormal sed rates. Patients with osteoarthritis and fibromyalgia, however, usually have normal sed rates. Some infections can also cause an abnormal sed rate; the test is not specific for any one disease.

Your doctor may also ask for another blood test to look for *rheumatoid factor.* Rheumatoid factor is an abnormal protein in the blood present in 70 to 80 percent of patients with rheumatoid arthritis. However, rheumatoid factor can also be present in otherwise normal persons.

Your doctor also may test for antinuclear antibody (ANA). Like the rheumatoid factor, ANA is an abnormal protein in the blood and is most commonly found with systemic lupus erythematosus. Lupus is a type of arthritis more commonly found in women, especially younger women. It can cause pain and fatigue, and may also cause internal organ problems, such as kidney disease, heart disease, or problems in the brain.

More than 90 percent of patients with lupus have a positive blood test for antinuclear antibody. However, the test can be positive in persons who do not have lupus or who have other, unrelated diseases. The ANA test is important, but there are usually other clues present as well for your doctor.

X Rays Show No Abnormality

X rays of the painful areas will show no abnormality, because the pain caused by fibromyalgia is in the soft tissues (muscles and tendons), which do not show up well on routine X rays. If you have another problem, such as arthritis, then there may be some abnormalities on the X rays to indicate what type of arthritis is present. Keep in mind that fibromyalgia does not cause X-ray changes.

It is important that you talk openly with your doctor in order to interpret the overall results of the total work-up, including the physical examination, laboratory testing, and X rays. This will allow you to have a good understanding of your problems and will provide the basis for your knowledge of the plan of treatment. At this time, be certain to ask any questions and even ask for printed information to read, if you feel the need.

Trust your doctor to decide which set of tests is best in your case to ensure no other medical problems are present. This can help you avoid extra testing that will add little to your diagnosis and only add expense. If there is one specific diagnosis you fear, such as cancer, be sure you tell your doctor. If you still do not feel comfortable with the diagnosis, talk to your doctor and have more testing. Or get a second opinion until you have peace of mind that the problem has been diagnosed correctly. At that time, proper treatment can begin.

Diagnostic Guidelines

Once other medical problems have been ruled out by laboratory tests and X rays, making the diagnosis of fibromyalgia may still be difficult. There are, however, some other guidelines and diagnostic criteria physicians use to determine the problem.

AMERICAN COLLEGE OF RHEUMATOLOGY CRITERIA FOR CLASSIFICATION OF FIBROMYALGIA

1. History of widespread pain
   Pain in left side of body
   Pain in right side of body
   Pain above waist
   Pain below waist
In addition, pain must be present in one of the following areas:
   Cervical spine (neck)
   Anterior chest (front of chest)
   Thoracic spine (middle back)
   Lumbar spine (lower back)
   Shoulder and buttock pain is considered as pain for each involved side.

2. Pain in eleven of eighteen tender or trigger point sites on palpation (see figure 2.1). Tender point sites are defined as follows (both sides, right and left):
   Occiput: at suboccipital muscle insertions
   Low cervical: at anterior aspects of intertransverse spaces at C5–C7
   Trapezius: at midpoint of upper border
   Supraspinatus: at origins, above scapular spine near medial border
   Second rib: at second costochondral junctions, just lateral to junctions on upper surfaces

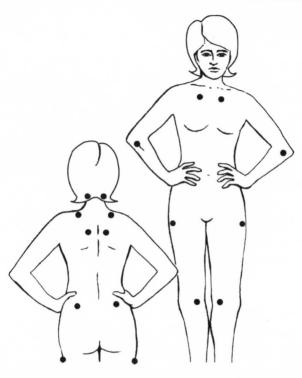

Figure 2.1. Trigger areas are tender points over the neck, shoulder blades, lower back, elbows, and knees or other areas. At least eleven of the eighteen trigger points are found to be painful in patients with fibromyalgia.

Lateral epicondyle (tennis elbow sites): 2 cm distal to epicondyles

Gluteal: in upper outer quadrants of buttocks in anterior fold of muscle

Greater trochanter: posterior to trochanteric prominence

Knee: at medial fat pad proximal to joint line

Patients have fibromyalgia if both criteria are satisfied. Widespread pain must have been present for three months.

The presence of a second clinical disorder does not exclude diagnosis of fibromyalgia.

Diagnosing Fibromyalgia

As your physician makes the proper diagnosis of fibromyalgia, there are three primary areas that will be considered:

1. Evaluating widespread pain
2. Evaluating trigger points
3. Eliminating other diseases

To be thorough with a diagnosis of fibromyalgia, the following six evaluations are important:

EVALUATE WIDESPREAD PAIN

As explained in chapter 1, patients tell of feeling pain "everywhere," or at least in so many places that it seems to be everywhere. The pain can be sharp, dull, aching, sticking, or pressurelike, or it may be difficult to characterize. The pain often comes from deep within the muscles or joints, as well as from the tendons and ligaments around the joints. Quite often people mistake this pain for a type of true arthritis because of the discomfort and stiffness.

However, the pain from fibromyalgia seems to be from *around* the joints more often than from the joints themselves. Unlike the pain that you may feel after engaging in exercise or a day of housecleaning, which goes away after you walk around, patients tell of pain being present twenty-four hours a day. It makes itself known in the morning on arising and stays all day, even worsening as the day goes on.

Pain is typically felt in the back, neck, arms, and legs, including the shoulders and elbows as well as the hips and buttocks. There may also be pain felt in the hands, wrists, knees,

ankles, and feet. Pain in the head and jaws can cause headaches or feelings of *temporomandibular joint syndrome*
(TMJ). This occurs when the temporomandibular joints (jaw
joints) and the muscle and ligaments that support them do not
work properly.

Pain is also commonly felt in the abdomen, along with
cramps, diarrhea, and constipation. Pain in the bladder area,
along with frequent urination, is common. Menstrual periods
may be much more painful than usual. Pain may be felt in the
chest and may be difficult to tell from pain due to heart disease.

The American College of Rheumatology found that almost
all fibromyalgia patients have widespread pain above the
waist, below the waist, on the right and left sides of their
bodies, and in the neck or back areas. Indeed, people with
fibromyalgia may have more pain receptors than others or
might be overly sensitive to everything. One patient said just
taking a warm bubble bath was a painful experience. The
symptom of widespread pain is important in making an accurate diagnosis and in telling the difference between fibromyalgia and other problems.

Understanding Acute and Chronic Pain Acute pain is important, because it brings to your attention a problem that
might cause damage to the body. Acute pain could be a tooth-
ache from a cavity, a broken bone, a headache from a sinus
infection, or a backache from a strain. Muscle pain, joint pain,
and pain in the stomach could all be acute signals of a potential problem. Some injuries can cause acute pain, such as the
pain associated with bursitis and tendinitis. Each of these
types of acute pain runs its course and disappears as the problem is relieved.

Surveys have shown that more than 70 percent of Americans have acute pain from headache at some time each year,
and more than 50 percent have backaches. These pains usu-

ally last a few days to weeks. When the problem is relieved, or the injury heals, the pain leaves. For example, acute back pain, the most common cause of loss of work except for the common cold, can come on suddenly and can be severe, but in more than 80 percent of cases it goes away in about two weeks.

Researchers consider acute pain that lasts one to six months longer than expected to be *chronic,* depending on the problem that causes the pain. For example, a back injury causes acute pain; if the pain is no better after three months, it is called chronic back pain. Pain that returns over and over for months or years can be considered chronic. Back pain that is severe and returns many times over one or more years is called chronic back pain. Pain from fibromyalgia is chronic; it lasts for at least three months.

Finding Underlying Problems Internal organ problems can cause chronic pain that may mimic the overall aching or throbbing muscle pain of fibromyalgia. If the pain is caused by kidney disease, stomach disease, or other internal organ abnormality, correcting the basic problem will remove the pain. Thus, it is necessary to find and treat any underlying causes of pain before starting treatment for what may seem to be pain from fibromyalgia.

For example, Colleen, a forty-seven-year-old woman, had chronic back pain for more than six months. She had been evaluated for ruptured lumbar disc, but the tests were negative. At that point, she read about fibromyalgia and immediately assumed that this was the proper diagnosis for her pain. However, further testing showed that she actually had a problem with gallbladder disease. After surgery on the gallbladder, her chronic back pain went away completely.

Another middle-aged woman came to our clinic with pain in the lower back and hip area that had lasted for months and had gradually become worse. When it began keeping her awake for several nights in a row, she became worried and sought further help. She was found to have cancer that had spread to the bones of the spine. After starting immediate treatment, she was free of pain.

EVALUATE TRIGGER POINTS

In 1990, the American College of Rheumatology established specific diagnostic criteria that require the presence of specific tender or trigger points that are painful to touch when pushed or palpated. In fact, these trigger points are key diagnostic features of the disease (see figure 2.1).

Trigger points, as discussed in chapter 1, are small, localized areas in muscles and tendons that are very tender to pressure in persons with fibromyalgia. These trigger areas are much more sensitive than other nearby areas. In fact, pressure on one of the trigger points with a finger causes pain that makes the person flinch or pull back. The actual size of a trigger point is usually very small, about the size of a penny. Trigger points are scattered over the neck, back, chest, elbows, hips, buttocks, and knees (see figure 2.1), and eleven or more of these are found in most patients with fibromyalgia.

In some conditions other than fibromyalgia, trigger-point pain may be felt in areas away from the actual tender trigger point. For example, pain may seem to travel down one or both legs when trigger areas are pushed in the lower back. This can mimic the pain of pressure on a nerve in the lower back from a ruptured disc, called *sciatica*.

When a physician tests trigger points for pain, he will also check *control points* or other nontender points on the body to make sure the person does not react to these as well, which would change the diagnosis. Some physicians use a special instrument, called a *doximeter* or *dolorimeter,* to apply just the right amount of pressure on trigger points.

ASK ABOUT FATIGUE

Fatigue has been estimated by researchers to be present at any one time in up to 25 percent of all of us. It can be mild and easily cured by getting extra rest and sleep. But fatigue, tiredness, and exhaustion can be prolonged (lasting more than one month) or chronic (lasting more than six months).

ASSESS YOUR LEVEL OF FATIGUE

Fatigue prevents you from doing normal activities and chores

Difficulty making plans due to unpredictable fatigue

Fatigue is unresolved after rest or at least eight hours of sleep

Fatigue interferes with work outside the home

Fatigue hinders relationship with family members and friends

Difficulty getting through the day because of fatigue

Fatigue prevents exercise or other activity

This loss of energy is the major complaint of most patients with fibromyalgia and may cause more limitation than the pain. Many patients tell us that if it were not for the fatigue, they could put up with the pain of fibromyalgia.

The fatigue associated with fibromyalgia severely limits daily activities. The tiredness may be especially bothersome in the morning and then improve after a few hours, only to return later in the day. There may be a window of time in each day when activities are tolerated after the morning fatigue wears off but before the afternoon fatigue hits again.

Patients tell of fatigue being most noticeable during activity, which causes immobility as the fatigue becomes more limiting. Fatigue can be even more severe following exercise—it may last days and be so worrisome that a person becomes sedentary.

Fatigue may be worse when a person is physically decondi-
tioned—out of shape. For example, if physical activity has
been avoided for a long enough period of time, muscle weakness or tiredness may by itself contribute to fatigue. Researchers have shown that most fibromyalgia patients have below
average fitness levels compared to other persons and when
these people do exercise, they complain of sore muscles without much effort. Many patients with fibromyalgia feel too
tired even to work, creating large disability and compensation
costs for their employers.

Another condition that can be hard to distinguish from
fibromyalgia and causes severe fatigue is *chronic fatigue syndrome* (CFS). In this condition, fatigue lasts more than six
months, interfering with daily activities both at home and
work, with no medical problem to explain it.

COMMON SYMPTOMS OF CHRONIC FATIGUE SYNDROME
Relentless fatigue
Memory and concentration problems
Sore throat
Swollen lymph nodes
Muscle and joint pains
Headaches
Poor sleep that is not restful
Exhaustion after exercise

A recent study from the American College of Rheumatology suggests that fibromyalgia and chronic fatigue syndrome may even overlap in the same person. With both
conditions, the fatigue and other symptoms seem to increase
after periods of high stress or physical exertion. Other studies
have indicated that many people who were initially diagnosed
as having chronic fatigue syndrome probably have fibromy-

algia. After some of these patients started the specific treatment for fibromyalgia, their symptoms lessened dramatically and their energy levels increased.

It may be hard to distinguish between fibromyalgia and chronic fatigue syndrome, as some patients with fibromyalgia tell of symptoms, listed above, that are similar to those of CFS. However, chronic fatigue syndrome patients usually have fever and swollen lymph nodes, and the onset of the problem is more sudden. Also, CFS patients don't usually have prominent trigger points of pain.

Your doctor can help you decide what your fatigue indicates, but other medical problems that cause fatigue need to be evaluated and eliminated.

INQUIRE ABOUT SLEEP DISTURBANCES

Almost all patients with fibromyalgia complain of sleep disturbances. They tell of waking up frequently during the night and feeling tired and unrefreshed during the day; many require more frequent rest periods during the day. Some researchers find that it may be the constant pain that interrupts sleep.

There is some evidence that sleep disturbances may be caused by an abnormality of deep sleep. Fibromyalgia patients show abnormal brain waveforms in deep sleep. Patients tell of feeling awake or in a shallow state of sleep throughout the night, instead of experiencing restful, deep-level sleep. Unfortunately, it is during the *delta,* or deep-level sleep, that the body does its repair work and replenishment. The hormone *somatostatin,* for example, which is produced in deep sleep and is vital for maintaining good muscle and other soft tissue health, has been found at low levels in fibromyalgia patients. If deep sleep is reduced over a long period of time, the body may have less ability to repair and replenish energy.

ASSESS SLEEP PROBLEMS

Many arousals during a night's sleep
Awakening in the middle of the night
Difficulty in getting to sleep
Reduction in total sleep time
Long awakenings (ten minutes or more) during sleep
Restless legs syndrome during sleep

EVALUATE STRESS LEVEL

Evaluating the patient's lifestyle and work habits to see if she is experiencing undue stress or uneasiness each day is an important factor in making a diagnosis. However, which came first: stress or fibromyalgia?

Doctors know that the stress of living with unending, throbbing, or stabbing pain and relentless fatigue can put the patient into overload, resulting in overwhelming feelings of nervousness and anxiety. But they are uncertain as to whether a stressful life brings about the fibromyalgia syndrome or whether having this disease leads to added stress. One study tested fibromyalgia patients on the Hospital Anxiety and Depression Index and a startling 92 percent of patients had a high score. Some consider fibromyalgia to be a psychosomatic illness in which psychological problems, such as depression, disappointment, and anxiety express themselves as physical symptoms, such as backache and sore muscles.

STRESSORS WITH FIBROMYALGIA

Physical stressors (the pain)
Social stressors (loss of friends and activities)
Work stressors (loss of job or difficulty working)
Family stressors (feeling of dependency on others)

No matter which came first, stress can add to problems of anger, distractibility, and irritability and can even lead to further physical changes, such as hypertension or cardiac problems.

ASSESS LEVEL OF STRESS
Various physical symptoms stemming from stress
Feeling overwhelmed day after day
Anxiety upon awakening
Impatient for no apparent reason
Unable to sleep soundly
Difficulty in concentrating on projects at home or work
Loss of interest or enjoyment in life
Easy to anger or frequent irritability
Changes in appetite (eating more or less food)

TEST FOR DEPRESSION
"I don't know if I'm depressed because I ache all over or because I am clinically depressed," Britt said. "I'm not used to being restricted in what I can do and feel caged in by this disease, as if it has a hold on me and won't let me feel free to move like I used to."

Britt told of depression lingering day after day, even when she had everything going for her. She had two healthy children and a husband who was supportive. "Every day I think that maybe this is the day that the sadness will lift. But after tossing and turning each night, I only awaken to more pain and sadness. Will it ever end?"

Again, which came first, fibromyalgia or depression? That question continues to puzzle many researchers, who have found that the two illnesses have similar characteristics. Many people with fibromyalgia are depressed. Conversely, depressed people often complain of inexplainable aches and pains along with fatigue and an inability to stay asleep at night. At some point researchers find depression present in the majority of fibromyalgia patients. In fact, *more than 25 percent* of patients do have depression when fibromyalgia is diagnosed.

When evaluating a patient, the doctor will talk about feelings of depression, as listed below.

COMMON SIGNALS OF DEPRESSION
Disturbances in sleep patterns
Loss of interest in usual activities
Weight loss or gain (more than 5 percent of body weight)
Fatigue
Impaired thinking
Thoughts of dying or suicide
Depressed thoughts or irritability
Mood swings
Staying at home all the time
Avoidance of special friends
Difficulty concentrating
Feelings of worthlessness or excessive or inappropriate guilt
Agitation or, in contrast, a general slowing of intentional
   bodily activity

Living with the constant pain and fatigue of fibromyalgia can bring about feelings of depression with hopelessness, uncontrollable tearfulness, loss of self-worth, and even suicidal thoughts. Some normal individuals may have one or more symptoms of depression at one time or another. Depression becomes a problem when symptoms begin to occur on a daily basis for a period of at least two weeks and are accompanied by other feelings, such as the fatigue, pain, and muscle aches.

Depression is a very complicated affliction and is not as easy to deal with as other worries and stressors mentioned in this chapter. Often, depression can stem from a biochemical imbalance or can be a symptom of an underlying ailment. Quite often professional help is needed to maintain, control, and cure depression. There are many excellent prescription drugs and many medical protocols that can assist greatly in controlling depression.

Fibromyalgia Can Be Discouraging

These are the most common feelings and signs of fibromyalgia your doctor may consider as he or she makes an accurate diagnosis. I know that these symptoms can be discouraging. The constant muscle pain and fatigue can make daily activities, such as standing, walking, sitting, and even coughing, unbearable. See Figure 2.2.

Pain and fatigue lead to inactivity. Because of the disrupted sleep patterns and failure to receive much needed restful sleep, the patient is fatigued even on arising. Daily fatigue can lead to personality changes. A once calm individual will now have a low frustration level, making it difficult to get along at home or work.

With the constant pain and feeling of exhaustion, it is no wonder the patient feels depressed. This in turn can lead to further feelings of discouragement and may create additional

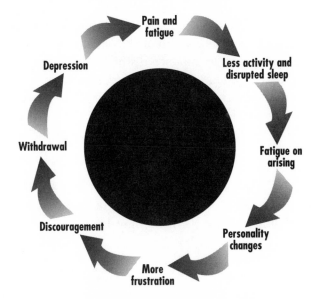

Figure 2.2. Cycle of depression with fibromyalgia

social problems and withdrawal from normal activities. Depression may worsen if certain medications, such as tranquilizers to aid with sleep, are used—especially if taken too frequently.

The 7-Step Treatment Program Does Work

The earlier the 7-Step Treatment Program is started, the better the chances are of improvement in a patient's symptoms. The program involves:

1. Experimenting with medications and treatments until a protocol that works is established.
2. Doing specific exercises to reduce muscle pain and increase strength and energy.
3. Learning ways to de-stress and alleviate anxiety at home and in the workplace.
4. Trying a complementary approach to reducing symptoms, including homeopathy, chiropractic, acupuncture, therapeutic touch, and biofeedback, among others.
5. Learning ways to enhance restful sleep and understanding the serotonin / fibromyalgia connection.
6. Starting a nutritional plan for healing using phytochemicals and antioxidants.
7. Understanding the importance of support for symptom relief.

The next seven chapters explain each of these important treatment modalities and if followed, will enable you to overcome the disabling effects of fibromyalgia.

3

STEP 1: START WITH MEDICAL TREATMENT

Jacqueline's experience was quite typical of most patients. She started out with excruciating pain upon arising one morning. She assumed this was a lingering symptom from the flu. Her doctor prescribed an over-the-counter pain medication and told her to drink plenty of fluids and get rest. This thirty-nine-year-old interior decorator told of staying in bed for two weeks, putting clients on hold, and farming her children out to friends while trying to get well.

"When I was no better two weeks later," she told me, "I knew I was up against something far worse than the winter flu." Jacqueline went from doctor to doctor, all of whom drew blood for lab work and took many X rays, but to no avail.

"When the last doctor sat me down and went over my chart, he looked at me and said, 'I cannot find anything wrong. You are a well person.' That did it! I knew I was not well, but I was determined to get well."

Jacqueline was diagnosed with fibromyalgia after going over her list of symptoms, including overall deep muscle pain, inability to sleep at night, depression, dizziness, irritable bowel syndrome, urinary frequency, painful menstrual cramps, and headaches. She was put on the 7-Step Treatment Program outlined in this book. While she is not cured, as there is no cure for this disease, she does have more good days than bad days and is able to function and do the things she wants to without debilitating symptoms.

If you have fibromyalgia and live with constant pain and fatigue, like millions of other sufferers, you have probably tried many ways to obtain relief. But to control the pain and other symptoms, you need a multidisciplinary approach. Each step described in the 7-Step Treatment Program is used in conjunction with the others and should be adapted to your lifestyle on a daily basis. Again, the steps will not cure the disease, but they will curb the symptoms.

Start with Moist Heat

Perhaps you have already tried a heating pad at times and found some relief for your aching muscles. I want you to carry this therapy further and use moist heat, twice daily, for ten to twenty minutes on areas of your body that have pain. Twice daily, every day without fail helps relax tense muscles, which makes exercising easier and relieves pain and more.

Because most patients complain of pain all over the body, the most effective and easy-to-use forms of moist heat are a warm shower, hot tub bath, whirlpool, or heated swimming pool. For example, it is easy to put a chair or stool (with rubber tips on the legs for safety) in the shower, then let the warm water permeate the back. Or, if you have access to a whirlpool bath or spa, use it twice daily. Some patients alternate the whirlpool and shower until they find one that is most effective. A warm bath may work for your overall pain, especially the legs and back, but with chronic pain, it may be difficult to sit and then get up from the tub.

If the pain is so intense that you cannot use the shower, whirlpool, or bathtub, then use warm, moist towels or a moist heating pad. Just put the moist towels on the back for a few minutes and change them for warm ones when they cool off. Another choice is hot packs, which can be purchased at a medical supply store. These are heated in hot water, wrapped in a towel, and placed on the back. Some packs are available that can be warmed in a microwave oven. These may be easier to use, but don't allow them to get too hot to touch.

INDIVIDUAL CHOICE IS IMPORTANT

Choose the form of moist heat that is most convenient and works best for you. Then plan to use it regularly—twice daily, every day. You may quickly find a reduction in pain that will last for a few minutes or hours. Mary Catherine told me emphatically that moist heat did nothing to relieve her pain, but upon questioning, she told me she only used it during her daily shower for ten minutes. Once she began a twice daily program, she experienced pain relief and was virtually sold on this part of the treatment program.

HELPFUL FORMS OF MOIST HEAT FOR FIBROMYALGIA PAIN

Heated swimming pool
Warm whirlpool or hot tub
Warm shower
Warm tub bath
Hot packs
Warm, moist towel or cloth
Moist heating pad

Add Medications

Certain medications are an effective part of the treatment program for fibromyalgia, along with the twice daily use of moist heat. Medications can provide much needed relief of the pain and deep, throbbing muscle aches. In our clinic, we encourage patients to use the lowest dosage possible of any medication and to find the medication that has the fewest side effects. Try to be patient. If pain relief is not experienced with the first medications you try, you and your physician may have to try other combinations.

If you notice unusual symptoms or side effects, stop taking the medication and talk to your doctor.

TRY ANTIDEPRESSANT MEDICATIONS

The most helpful medicines are from a group of prescription drugs used for years mainly to treat depression, specifically tricyclic and tetracyclic antidepressant drugs. This is an example of medicines that can be used for more than one purpose. The rationale for their use is twofold—most increase the time spent in stage 4 sleep, and they increase the amount of serotonin in the central nervous system, which has a calming effect (see page 60).

It may take two or three weeks before any improvement is shown. In fact, it may be necessary to try more than one antidepressant (one at a time) to find the most effective one. About 30 to 60 percent of patients find these medicines improve the symptoms of pain and depression.

Side effects are usually few if lower doses of the medicines are used. The most common side effects are drowsiness (which may help improve the quality of sleep when taken at night), dryness in the mouth, constipation (which is usually not serious), or occasional difficulty in urination. Less common side effects are dizziness, blurred vision, rapid heart rate, or confusion. If you also take other medication, check with your doctor to make sure there are no unwanted problems from the combination of drugs.

SOME COMMONLY USED
ANTIDEPRESSANT MEDICATIONS IN TREATING FIBROMYALGIA

TRADE NAME	GENERIC NAME
Elavil	amitriptyline
Norpramin	desipramine
Pamelor	nortriptyline
Paxil	paroxetene
Prozac	fluoxetine
Sinequan	doxepin
Tofranil	imipramine
Zoloft	sertraline

NONSTEROIDAL ANTI-INFLAMMATORY DRUGS

Often, nonsteroidal anti-inflammatory drugs (NSAIDs) are given to patients with fibromyalgia. Since there is little inflammation with the disease, these drugs usually are not very effective. But these medications can also have some pain-relieving *(analgesic)* effect that may give relief at times. If you don't find relief from pain after about two weeks, try a different nonsteroidal anti-inflammatory drug or an acetaminophen (such as Tylenol), which is not a NSAID and is well tolerated by asthmatics and people with gastrointestinal problems.

SOME COMMON NONSTEROIDAL ANTI-INFLAMMATORY DRUGS

TRADE NAME	GENERIC NAME
Advil	ibuprofen
Aleve	naproxen
Anaprox	naproxen
Ansaid	flurbiprofen
Aspirin products	acetylsalicyclic acid
Clinoril	sulindac
Daypro	oxaprozin
Disalcid	salsalate
Dolobid	diflunisal

TRADE NAME	GENERIC NAME
Feldene	piroxicam
Indocin	indomethacin
Lodine	etodolac
Magan	magnesium salicylate
Meclomen	meclofenamate
Monogesis	salsalate
Motrin	ibuprofen
Nalfon	fenoprofen
Naprosyn	naproxen
Orudis	ketoprofen
Oruvail	ketoprofen
Relafen	nabumetone
Salflex	salsalate
Tolectin	tolmetin
Trilisate	choline magnesium trisalicylate
Voltaren	diclofenac sodium
Zorprin	zero-order release aspirin

If these drugs give relief, they can be used for a long period of time, but you must always watch for side effects, especially for any upset stomach, since peptic ulcers are a possibility. Other serious side effects include dark, sticky bowel movements and blood in the stool. About 1 percent of those who take these NSAIDs for six months or longer have blood in their stool.

You will need to have a blood test taken every few months to check for side effects. If you have any questions, talk to your doctor before you continue to take any NSAIDs.

SOME OF THE MOST COMMON SIDE EFFECTS OF NSAIDS
Abdominal pain
Abnormal liver tests (blood tests)
Allergic or unusual reactions
Anemia (lower hemoglobin)

Asthma in those allergic
Blurred vision (occasional)
Confusion
Constipation
Decreased platelet count (can affect bleeding)
Depression
Diarrhea
Difficulty sleeping
Diminished effect of diuretics
Dizziness
Fatigue
Gastritis
Headaches
Heartburn
Hypertension (increased blood pressure)
Impaired thinking (uncommon, but occurs at times in older
    people)
Indigestion
Intestinal bleeding
Itching
Lowered white cells in blood count
Meningitis-like illness (rare)
Mouth ulcers
Palpitations
Peptic ulcers
Rash
Renal (kidney) failure
Sleepiness
Sodium retention with edema (swelling)
Sun sensitivity
Tinnitus (ringing in the ears)

CORTISONE-TYPE DRUGS

Cortisone-type drugs are almost never given regularly by
mouth to fibromyalgia patients, as the side effects of long-

term use are not worth the benefits. On the other hand, local injections of a cortisone derivative into a painful trigger point can be used. This type of injection is usually combined with a local anesthetic and can give good relief from pain at the particular trigger point that may last from weeks to months (see page 55).

MUSCLE RELAXANTS

Many patients find temporary relief for back and neck pain with such muscle relaxants as cyclobenzaprine (Flexeril), chlorzoxazone (Parafon Forte), methocarbamol (Robaxin), or carisoprodol (Soma). The benefit of muscle relaxants is that they can be used as needed, since they usually give rapid relief that lasts for a few hours. If they don't, then they should be eliminated.

Side effects of muscle relaxants are usually not serious. The most common side effect is drowsiness.

NONNARCOTIC PAIN MEDICATIONS

Two nonnarcotic prescription pain medicines, Toradol or Ultram, may give relief for hours and can be used when needed. It is important to be sure, however, that your activity level is improving when these medications are used for treating fibromyalgia pain. There is no real advantage in simply killing the pain and remaining inactive.

NARCOTIC PAIN MEDICATIONS

Narcotic prescription pain medicines are not recommended for regular use in the treatment of fibromyalgia pain, since narcotics can be habit-forming, and it is likely that there will be a need to find a better long-term solution for pain control. Narcotics can aggravate depression, which can be a part of the fibromyalgia patient's problems.

Narcotic pain medications commonly cause constipation if taken regularly.

MEDICINES FOR RESTFUL SLEEP

Prescription sleeping pills can also aggravate depression and often don't give excellent results in most patients. Your doctor can help you decide if they would be helpful in your own situation.

Recently, melatonin has been cited in the media as a breakthrough for the treatment of various sleep disorders. It has been referred to as the hormone of darkness, as its secretion is activated almost immediately after exposure to darkness. Melatonin induces sleepiness and, in some cases, gives a sensation of well-being and moderate elation. Several studies have shown it to be effective in alleviating jet lag and certain types of insomnia. However, its effect has not been studied in patients with fibromyalgia.

Large doses of melatonin may cause headaches and abdominal cramps. When given to patients with depression, melatonin can increase self-ratings of depression, and paradoxically, increase the degree of insomnia. Although melatonin has been sold at health food stores for several years, its purity cannot be reliably confirmed and over-the-counter tablets may contain up to ten times the level of the hormone normally produced by the body during sleep.

Even though it is widely used, melatonin has not yet been approved or even classified by the Food and Drug Administration (FDA); it is still viewed as an experimental drug. No conclusive studies have been done on humans regarding its possible long-term side effects.

Combining Treatment with Medications

In our clinic, we find that a combination of heat and exercise, along with one of the antidepressant medications and the most effective nonsteroidal anti-inflammatory drug, gives the best relief in the deep muscle pain. I will tell you up front that choosing the medications does require some trial and error. However, it is important that you patiently try the available medications in each group to be sure you have the best chance for success in pain control and increased activity.

Minimize Food and Drug Interactions

There are preventive measures you can take to ensure the least possible interaction between food and the drugs you take. Some medications must be taken immediately following a meal; others must be taken on an empty stomach. Some medications cannot be mixed with alcohol or the end result can be deadly. If you drink alcohol with an antidepressant, for example, the results can be excessive intoxication. Alcohol taken with a muscle relaxant depresses brain activity, and alcohol with a hypnotic / sedative (sleeping pill) causes over-sedation and can even be fatal. Carefully follow your pharmacist's instructions on each prescription and over-the-counter medication you take, and be sure to contact your physician if you have any questions concerning medication and possible reactions.

Below are descriptions of just a few of the drugs that may be given and their interaction with food.

ACETAMINOPHEN (TYLENOL). Take on an empty stomach as food delays absorption.

ASPIRIN. Take with food as medication may cause gastrointestinal upset. Long-term use may cause gastrointestinal bleeding and contribute to iron deficiency anemia. Should not be used by people prone to bleeding or deficient in vitamin K. Diet recommendations: For long-term use increase food sources of vitamin C (oranges, orange juice, other citrus fruit, green leafy vegetables, cantaloupe, strawberries, and broccoli).

AMITRIPTYLINE (ELAVIL). Take with food. Diet recommendations: Avoid alcohol. May cause an increase in appetite for carbohydrate-containing foods. May cause dry mouth.

IBUPROFEN (ADVIL, MOTRIN). Take with meals or milk. Diet recommendations: Avoid alcohol. Watch for nausea or indigestion or other abdominal discomfort.

NAPROXEN (ALEVE). Take with meals. Diet recommendations: Avoid alcohol. Watch for nausea, indigestion, or other abdominal discomfort.

Other Medical Modalities for Treating Pain

LOCAL INJECTIONS

Local injections, combined with a local anesthetic (a low dose of a cortisone derivative or corticosteroid), can be helpful when there are painful trigger points. Within a few days, there is often relief of pain from the localized trigger point and surrounding areas, with relief often lasting weeks at a time. This treatment is especially good when there are one or two trigger points causing major pain and limited movement. Also, if there is improvement in many areas but one or two painful areas remain, then local injection can be very helpful.

There are usually no serious side effects, and there should be no significant problems from an occasional local injection of these areas of tissue pain. The cortisone dose should have little effect on the rest of the patient's body.

OTHER INJECTIONS FOR PAIN

There are several types of injections available other than those used on trigger points. Injections around the spine in specific areas (epidural injections, facet joint injections, and nerve block) using a local anesthetic and a cortisone derivative may give pain relief that lasts for weeks or months. If this has positive results, the injections may be repeated after several months. Sometimes, stopping the pain temporarily may have a lasting effect on the chronic pain.

ULTRASOUND

Ultrasound uses sound waves that are applied to the muscles, tendons, and other soft tissues of the back. This may help relaxation, decrease inflammation, and improve pain in tender points. It is more commonly used for acute back pain and other similar situations than for chronic pain. It can be done properly by your physical therapist and continued if it gives relief.

TENS

Transcutaneous Electrical Nerve Stimulation (TENS) uses electrical stimulation for pain relief from many different causes. Electrical impulses sent to certain nerves block the messages of pain being sent by other nerves from the painful area. These impulses might also cause the body to release *endorphins,* which are natural pain relievers produced by the body.

The person wears a unit, a stimulator and battery, usually on a belt. Electrical wires from the stimulator attach to electrodes held by adhesive, usually a patch, on the skin. The electrodes are placed in the area of pain but may need to be tried at different locations to get the best relief.

The TENS unit can be used continuously or only as needed

for the pain. Usually there will be a trial of about one month
to see the effect on pain.

LONG-TERM NARCOTIC INJECTION
In unusual cases of some chronic pain, surgery can be used to
insert a catheter for long-term use of drugs, such as narcotics,
for pain control. A device called a *port* is installed, usually on
the abdomen, which allows injections of medication as often
as needed. A pump can also be installed through surgery to
allow medication (such as morphine) to be delivered continuously for additional pain relief.

COMPREHENSIVE PAIN CLINIC
As discussed in chapter 9, a comprehensive pain clinic may be
useful, but only after you have tried the 7-Step Treatment
Program and are still living with pain each day.

Read the criteria for finding a qualified pain clinic on pages
149 to 151 and with your doctor's consultation, choose one
that best suits your particular needs.

Trial and Error to Wellness

In short, there is hope to treat fibromyalgia's symptoms. While
there is no quick fix, you can find success with treatment using
a trial-and-error procedure. That is, you must work with your
physician and try various medications and medical or complementary treatments to find the ones that will help. This will
take some time as you sort through the options, but you will
see greater benefits in the long run with symptom control,
including pain management and less fatigue.

4

STEP 2:
EXERCISE DAILY FOR
MOBILITY AND ENERGY

Janet spoke of living with the symptoms of fibromyalgia for five years, traveling from doctor to doctor, complaining of widespread pain, tenderness at specific tender points, muscular weakness, and an overall flulike exhaustion. "I think most of them thought that I was this stereotypical hysterical female, but I knew differently. I knew that something was terribly wrong with me," she said.

This thirty-four-year-old mother and homemaker was an avid runner before she had children. "In college I used to run several miles each day before classes," she continued. "Then I started my career and family, and I never found time to exercise. Now I couldn't exercise if I wanted to."

This young woman is characteristic of so many patients, that is, most are aerobically unfit and not engaging in any regular exercise. Research has found that fibromyalgia patients are more than *75 to 80 percent below average in fitness* compared with age- and gender-matched subjects of the general population.

I have heard a myriad of excuses from patients as to why they avoid exercise, including:

"How can I exercise? I can hardly walk to my car each morning."

"Sure I'd exercise if only I had some energy."

"Exercise frightens me. What if it makes this disease worse?"

"I tried to walk around the block the other day, and it left me exhausted."

"There's no way this tired body can exercise. I can hardly make dinner."

"If I could ever sleep all night without tossing and turning, then maybe I'd feel like exercising."

"If you could cure me of fibromyalgia, I'd be glad to start exercising."

Exercise Is Essential for Muscle Strength and Flexibility

Both as a doctor and as someone who exercises daily, I know that a regular exercise program is essential to keep muscles strong and flexible, to control weight, and to stay active in other areas of life. Aerobic exercise particularly has also been shown to improve symptoms and restore muscle strength in patients with fibromyalgia. In fact, exercise and activity allow patients to have some control over the disease and the amount of pain they feel.

If you want to reduce your pain and get more energy, you will have to start exercising. Lou was the most resistant patient I'd ever treated when it came to moving around. Even though she had successfully followed the other steps in the treatment program, she refused to exercise.

"When I think of moving my legs and arms, all that comes to mind is pain, pain, and more pain," Lou said strongly. "And I'm sick and tired of living with pain."

It took three months to convince Lou that even though the pain wouldn't go away immediately, she would begin to notice a difference in her pain threshold within several weeks of starting her exercise program. And at her six-month visit, Lou found that exercise was the missing link in her treatment. Six months before, this fifty-two-year-old woman could hardly climb up onto the examining table. Now Lou was lifting her arms and stretching down to the floor—without pain.

In our clinic, we see patients who are able to see and feel great improvement with managing symptoms by maintaining a regular exercise program. Not only does exercise slow down the heart-racing adrenaline associated with stress, but those with fibromyalgia experience the added benefit of boosting levels of endorphins (proteins that reduce feelings of pain and induce euphoria), helping to relieve low-grade depression, and also helping them to receive restful sleep.

Exercise Boosts Serotonin Levels

Serotonin is a neurotransmitter in the brain that scientists have found to be related to fibromyalgia. (Neurotransmitters are chemicals that send specific messages from one brain cell to another.) While only a small percentage of all serotonin (1 to 2 percent) is located in the brain, this neurotransmitter is believed to play a vital role in mediating moods.

Studies have found that too much stress can lead to permanently low levels of serotonin, which can create aggression. When serotonin levels are increased in the brain, it is associated with a calming, anxiety-reducing effect, and in some cases, with drowsiness. Also, a stable serotonin level in the brain is associated with a positive mood state or feeling good over a period of time. Lack of exercise and inactivity can aggravate low serotonin levels.

It also appears that women may have a greater sensitivity to the changes in this brain chemical. Mood swings during the menstrual cycle, menopause, or following the birth of a child

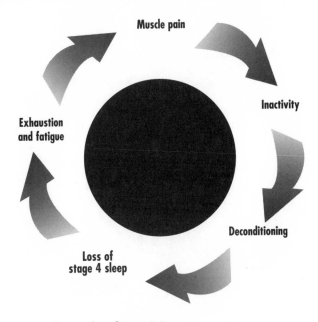

Muscle pain

Inactivity

Exhaustion and fatigue

Deconditioning

Loss of stage 4 sleep

Figure 4.1. The cycle of inactivity

may be induced by the action of hormones on neurotransmitters.

Various factors can have a positive effect on serotonin levels, including sunlight, certain carbohydrate foods, some hormones, and exercise. Not only does exercise act as nature's tranquilizer, helping to boost serotonin levels in the brain, but studies have shown that exercise also triggers the release of epinephrine and norepinephrine, which are known to boost alertness. For those who feel stressed-out frequently, exercise will help to desensitize your body to stress.

Before starting an exercise program, most patients experience a cycle of inactivity that usually begins with muscle pain and leads to inactivity, poor physical conditioning, and disrupted stage 4 (delta) sleep. This vicious cycle can be halted with increased exercise and fitness.

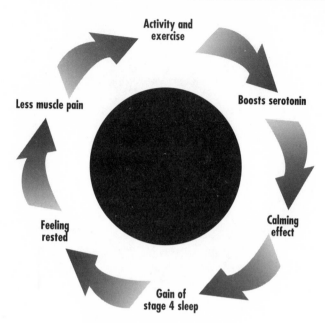

Figure 4.2. The cycle of activity

Exercise: Safe and Necessary

Until recently, many researchers felt that exercise might exacerbate fibromyalgia's symptoms or accelerate the disease; thus, physicians encouraged patients to seek rest, not activity. But more recent scientific tests are conclusive in determining that, for most patients, range of motion, strengthening, and aerobic conditioning exercises are safe and necessary.

Most patients have a reduced quality of life, which can be the result of impaired endurance. Because of this, exercise is one of the first modes of treatment I encourage patients to undertake in order to reduce pain, improve endurance for physical activities, improve cardiovascular fitness, and cope with life's stressors, including their disease, in a more accepting manner. In fact, I have found that most patients can push themselves to exercise, even if they have not exercised for years and are in some pain.

If you are considering undertaking the recommended exercise program described in this book, I urge you to consult first with your physician to determine the type and intensity of the exercise or activity.

BENEFITS OF REGULAR EXERCISE FOR FIBROMYALGIA PATIENTS

- Improves sense of well-being
- Strengthens bones
- Strengthens muscles
- Gives range of motion to painful muscles and joints
- Increases aerobic capacity
- Improves quality of sleep
- Stimulates growth hormone secretion
- Burns calories and makes weight control easier
- Increases cardiovascular health
- Reduces anxiety levels and depression
- Secretes endorphins or "happy hormones"
- Improves outlook on life
- Relieves stress associated with a chronic disease
- Increases energy
- Places the responsibility of healing in the hands of the patient

Different Types of Exercise

As you begin your exercise program, you will focus on three different types of exercise:

Range-of-motion or stretching exercises. These involve moving a joint as far as it will go (without pain) or through its full range of motion. The range-of-motion exercises or stretching will help you maintain flexibility in your muscle groups.

Endurance or conditioning exercises. When you increase your endurance threshold with cardiovascular forms of exercise, such as walking, biking, or swimming, you will not only strengthen your muscles, but also condition your body and build coordination and endurance.

Strengthening exercises. These exercises help to build strong muscles and tendons needed to support your joints. I recommend cautiously performing strength training using either resistance machines, resistance bands, or free weights (handheld weights that are not part of a machine).

Range-of-Motion or Stretching Exercises

Flexibility, the ability to move your joints through their full range of motion, is one of the key elements of fitness, along with cardiovascular endurance and muscle strength. Yet most patients have become inflexible because they have avoided exercise due to fatigue. This condition varies from one person to the next, as one patient may be flexible in her spine yet stiff in her shoulders. Another person may be able to bend down and touch the floor yet not be able to bend from side to side without pain and stiffness. Being flexible also helps protect you from joint injury, and the best way to get this protection is through stretching before activity or exercise.

More than anyone, sedentary people need the relief from muscle tension and stiffness that stretching provides. When done correctly, stretching feels good and is healing. Not only does a stretched muscle experience an increase in muscle tone, mobility, and greater circulation along with a marked decrease in pain, but also is less likely to be injured. Improper or excessive stretching, however, may actually increase the likelihood of injury—something you want to avoid with a chronic pain disease.

SEEK INSTRUCTION FROM A PHYSICAL THERAPIST

Because fibromyalgia's symptoms are physiologic in nature, you may want to seek instruction from a licensed physical therapist. These professionals have a background in anatomy and *kinesiology* (study of movement) allowing them to develop specific stretching and strengthening programs for your specific needs.

Physical therapy can enable you to regain control of your illness as you focus on lifestyle changes rather than on the chronic dysfunction. Proper posture, which your physical therapist will help you with, allows efficient muscle function, thus avoiding undue fatigue and pain. The slow stretching exercises on pages 168 to 178, performed *after* the application of moist heat, will improve muscle flexibility and reduce muscle tension.

Be sure that symptom relief modalities, such as heat and gentle massage, are only used for brief periods of time and in preparation for active exercise.

BEGIN A STRETCHING ROUTINE

Your stretching routine should be specific and include all the major muscle groups, including shoulders, hips, pelvis, buttocks, thighs, and calves.

Begin your stretching regime with five minutes of walking in place until your body warms up. This enables sore, tight muscles to loosen up. Then work at stretching one muscle at a time, holding your stretch for at least thirty to sixty seconds. A word of caution: Avoid overdoing this, as you don't want to add more damage to your aching muscles.

While it is important to get to the point where you can do stretches daily, you must make a conscious effort to do the exercise correctly in order to obtain optimal benefit. It is better to do only a few stretches correctly than to hurry through them and risk injury.

Again, if stretching is done right, it should feel good. If you experience pain, check with your physician or physical therapist. The goal of stretching is to *decrease* pain and immobility, not increase it.

For more information about how to stretch properly, check with a physical therapist in your area. You can seek recommendations from your physician or contact the Private Practice Section, American Physical Therapy Association, 1101 17th Street, NW, Suite 1000, Washington, DC 20036. Phone (202) 457-1115.

Endurance or Conditioning Exercises

Recent studies have shown that aerobic fitness is a factor in regulating the altered sleep patterns characteristic of fibromyalgia. Tests have been done on patients, comparing aerobic exercise to range-of-motion or stretching exercise. While both were found beneficial, patients who performed aerobic exercises regularly showed greater improvement in quality of sleep and trigger-point pain thresholds.

In our clinic, we find that some of the best types of conditioning exercises for patients are walking and water exercises. When performed regularly, these cardiovascular exercises can strengthen muscles and help to relieve depression. And then there's the added benefit of aerobic exercise: It not only challenges the heart and lungs, but by sustaining an elevated heart rate, it will enable you to burn fat and control your weight. Maintaining a normal weight is important for people with any type of chronic pain. It enables you to have more energy and relieves you of unnecessary pressure on painful muscles.

Again, your warm-up should include walking in place for

several minutes along with stretching your muscles and joints in full range of motion. Use the suggested exercises on page 168.

CHECK YOUR PULSE

During exercise, it is important to take your pulse periodically. You can do this by placing your finger (not your thumb) on the artery on the side of your windpipe (your carotid pulse) or on the thumb side of the wrist. Slow your pace during your workout and count your pulse rate for ten seconds. Multiply this number by six to get your total pulse for one minute.

Your pulse rate should stay within your target heart range during exercise. This range can be found using the chart below. Or, you can compute this yourself by subtracting your age from 220 and multiplying the number you get by 60 percent. This gives you the low end of your range. Now subtract your age from 220 and multiply this number by 80 percent to get the high end of your range. If your total pulse rate is higher than your target range, you should slow down. If the pulse rate is lower than the range, you may choose to work harder. Some inactive patients will find that their pulse rate will increase with very little exercise or activity.

ESTIMATED TARGET HEART RANGES FOR VARIOUS AGES DURING EXERCISE

Age	Low	High	Age	Low	High
20–21	120	162	54–55	102	132
22–25	114	156	56–57	96	132
26–27	114	156	58–59	96	126
28–29	114	156	60–62	96	126
30–35	114	150	63–65	96	126
36	108	150	66	90	126
37–44	108	144	67–70	90	120
45	108	138	71–74	90	120
46–51	102	138	75	90	114
52–53	102	132	76–78	84	114

The chart on the previous page provides an estimate for the low and high end of your target heart rate. During exercise, find your pulse rate for one minute as directed above. This total rate should fit within the recommended range for safe exercise.

START WITH WALKING

Walking may be the best all-around exercise for people with fibromyalgia. It can be done by almost anyone at any time and at any place . . . and it's free! I've seen patients improve their symptoms of pain, stiffness, and fatigue by simply adding fifteen to twenty minutes of walking to their daily routine. Because this low-impact form of exercise is less likely to cause an injury than running or aerobics, it is preferred by many as a safe way to become conditioned.

Beatrice, a forty-four-year-old woman who has lived with fibromyalgia for seven years, said that walking boosts her spirits, especially on days when pain and fatigue seem to overwhelm her. "I love to walk and hike in our neighborhood," she said. "On really bad days when my symptoms flair, I make myself walk anyway. I take a cane to give me added support and allow more time."

Not only will walking tone the muscles in your legs and upper body, but it will increase your metabolism and help with weight management. For women, walking offers a much needed bonus, as it increases bone density, which helps prevent a common disease of aging, *osteoporosis* (brittle bones).

You may wonder about those patients who can barely stand up, much less begin a walking program. In my experience, most people can start this program by making small goals. For example, if you have great pain during movement, begin by walking indoors from room to room for five minutes. As you progress in strength, walk around your house or apartment; then walk around your block. Your pace will depend on your capability and pain threshold, but by taking small steps, most people can achieve an adequate level of fitness. Remember, walking some is better than not walking at all.

Many prefer an indoor treadmill that can be used at home, so bad weather is no excuse, and it can be done anytime, day or night.

REFRESH WITH WATER EXERCISES

Perhaps more than any other conditioning exercise, my patients tell of enjoying water exercises the most. Forty-one-year-old Robert said that water exercise is almost as refreshing as a nap. "I can be having a rough day, feeling sorry for myself and aching all over, then I go over to the swimming pool at my apartment complex and get in the water. Something magical happens while exercising. In just minutes, I feel more optimistic and less pain. It works wonders for me and even helps me to sleep more soundly."

Numerous studies have been done recently on the benefits of water exercise to people with arthritic diseases. The findings are consistent with what Robert claims, that is, water exercise is a perfect no-impact activity that just about anyone can do without injury or stress to an aching joint. Most people report feeling better after a water exercise routine. Stretching or even walking in water is particularly comforting as the buoyancy of the water supports your body, putting less pressure on trigger points.

There are water vests and life jackets you can purchase that allow you to exercise in water without fear of going under. An aqua vest will place you in a near weightless position so you can stretch and strengthen muscles easily.

Most YMCA programs offer aquatic classes, teaching you the range-of-motion and aerobic exercises that can be done in water. Often, special classes are offered specifically for people with arthritis, and the trained instructors can assist you in designing a water exercise program for your specific fibromyalgia needs.

Strengthening Exercises

For those over the age of forty the muscle pain and weakness associated with fibromyalgia present an even greater problem. Studies show that muscle strength naturally levels off at midlife. There is good news, though; resistance or weight training can offset this muscle decline and help build strength in aching muscles.

Studies have found that weight training brings about marked improvement for patients, although over the past decades, a greater emphasis has been placed on aerobics than weight training for pain relief. However, aerobics is a conditioning exercise for the heart and is not designed for developing muscle size. I have seen many patients become discouraged when, after weeks of aerobic exercise, they don't feel any lessening in deep muscle pain. That is why in order to strengthen your muscles, it is important to supplement your exercise routine with weight training.

COMMON MISCONCEPTIONS OF WEIGHT TRAINING

"I don't want to look like a football player," one petite woman said after we set her up with a qualified personal trainer to help with a resistance training program. Many people still associate weights with building bulky muscles, but this is not the case. Let's look at some of the common misconceptions of weight training.

1. Weight lifting is dangerous. False. If done with proper technique, lifting weights is a very safe way to tone the body.

2. If you stop, muscles will turn to fat. False. This is physiologically impossible. If you stop weight lifting, the muscles will lose size and tone, and any excess calories will be deposited as fat.

3. Women will get big muscles. False. Women produce less testosterone than men and build muscle size less rapidly. It takes years of hard work and proper diet to obtain large muscles.

4. Strength training means using heavy equipment. False. Resistance bands can be used as strength training. Other ways to strength-train include using isometrics, free weights, or even water-resistant exercises.

5. You must start with heavy weights. False. You should *not* begin with heavy weights. A good rule of thumb is to start with a weight you can easily lift ten times with the last two repetitions being increasingly difficult. For some people this is only one to two pounds; others can start at fifteen to twenty pounds, depending on their muscle strength. As your muscles gain strength and if there is no pain, increase the weights in one- to two-pound increments.

6. The theory "no pain, no gain" is true for strength training. False. If your muscles are very sore, do not use resistance training until you are relatively pain-free. Strength training may not be appropriate for every patient; check with your doctor for approval.

7. You will get high blood pressure. False. Weight training does not cause high blood pressure. Some people strain their body and hold their breath during a lift, which results in a temporary increase of blood pressure. However, holding your breath is *never recommended* during weight training.

8. You will become bulky and inflexible. False. It is important to supplement your weight training with a stretching routine to stay flexible.

9. Lifting weights helps me spot-reduce specific areas of my body. False. Exercise is not site-specific; you must exercise the total body to achieve maximum results.

10. The benefits are many. True. Increased strength, improved muscle tone, enhanced athletic performance, increased bone, tendon, and ligament strength, injury prevention, and improved body image are all benefits of weight training. For women, weight training can play a significant role in reducing osteoporosis, as bones need regular resistance to stay strong. And age is no factor with weight training; the muscles of older people are just as responsive as those of younger people.

GETTING STARTED WITH WEIGHT TRAINING

As you plan your resistance program, you should lift at least two to three times per week, with at least forty-eight to seventy-two hours between sessions for muscles to recover. Select an exercise for each of the body parts: legs (calves, quads, and hamstrings), abdomen, back, chest, shoulders, and arms (biceps and triceps).

One problem with weight training: Neglecting to exercise a body part can lead to imbalances in your body. Proper form is critical, whether you use free weights or machines. To ensure proper form and technique, it would be advantageous to use a qualified personal trainer the first few sessions. Your physician can help you find a trainer, if needed.

Initially, you should start out using very light weights or resistance of only one to two pounds, concentrating more on form. You can gradually add weight as long as proper form is maintained. Once you find a comfortable weight, you should stay with that weight for one to two sets of ten repetitions per body part, taking one to three minutes between sets to ensure a good quality workout.

TRY CIRCUIT TRAINING

Another way to weight-train is called circuit training. This is a group of machines that exercise all the body parts. You may be less likely to get injured using machines than using free weights. Free weights also can take months of practice before you become adept at sophisticated lifting techniques.

Heat or Ice?

All of the exercises described in this chapter will be much more effective and you will be more comfortable doing them if, before beginning, you take a warm shower for five to ten minutes to help you loosen up. You can even begin stretching while in the shower. After you complete the exercise program, take another warm shower if you have pain.

Some people feel more relief when they use ice packs instead of moist heat. A plastic bag or ice bag filled with ice can be applied to the painful area for about ten minutes. Don't place ice directly on your skin. Some patients get the most relief when they alternate treatments—moist heat then ice pack. Choose the combination that works best for you.

Remember—those who do their exercises regularly have a much higher chance of improving their symptoms. Do your exercises on good days and bad days, even when it is inconvenient. Once you are used to exercising, the time needed will be minimal and the rewards will be great. People frequently tell me that when they do their exercises they feel much better—and when they skip them, they feel worse. Exercises work!

Exercise Cautions for Fibromyalgia Patients

While an ongoing, daily exercise program will help you to see the short-term results of increased mobility and decreased pain, it can take months to build strong muscles. You can make the muscles that support your aching joints stronger and more flexible, but it takes time.

It is important to set personal exercise goals as you begin the prevention plan. Your goal may be to exercise for five minutes each day for the first two weeks. Once you get in the habit of doing this, then increase this exercise goal by another five minutes until you reach the suggested fifteen to twenty minutes or more of conditioning exercises, four to five times a week. Be sure you include a warm-up (walking or light jogging in place) before you begin your workout, then move to stretching, conditioning, and a few minutes of cooldown, which can include walking around while stretching your muscles again.

5

STEP 3:
DE-STRESS YOUR LIFE

D octor, I do apologize for being here, for I know you think I'm crazy." I hear this all the time. The varying, nonspecific symptoms of fibromyalgia, along with no scientific means to diagnose the disease, makes it is easy to feel as if the condition is imagined or in one's head. But research has shown again and again that fibromyalgia is not a psychiatric illness, even though millions of fibromyalgia patients have psychiatric symptoms, including depression, anxiety, and related disorders.

There is great speculation that stress or an inability to handle life's daily stressors may play an important part in the ebb and flow of fibromyalgia symptoms. Some researchers have tried to correlate high levels of stress with susceptibility to viral infection, while others have speculated that fibromyalgia could be viewed as "associated with dysregulation of the stress system."

If you are like many of my patients with fibromyalgia, perhaps you do not know how to de-stress your life so that these additional symptoms don't become a permanent fixture. Brenda, a middle-aged mother of teenage sons, tells of feeling nervous and having frequent panic attacks, especially when her fibromyalgia symptoms flair. But it may not be the fibromyalgia that is causing this excess anxiety; Brenda also tells of being "on call" for everyone in her family in addition to working part-time and caring for her aging parents.

Brenda's enslavement to pleasing those around her without thought of her own health and well-being is shared by many today, especially women. It can cause problems when you have a chronic disease and are faced with a new set of limitations. Fortunately, these limitations can be lessened, if you take active steps to get your life and priorities in order.

Is There a Fibromyalgia Personality?

While in the past, some observations have described a stereotypical obsessive compulsive, perfectionistic fibromyalgia personality, current studies do not support this observation. Using standard diagnostic criteria, researchers found that only 5 to 6 percent of fibromyalgia patients could be classified as having obsessive-compulsive disorder (OCD). Using psychological testing, these researchers found that approximately one-third of fibromyalgia patients are psychologically disturbed, one-third have a chronic pain profile, and one-third are "normal."

I feel that it is important to understand that patients with fibromyalgia will always score high on the hypochondriasis and hysteria scales of these tests since such scales are scored by summing the patient's physical complaints. It makes sense that if a well person were in constant pain and could not achieve restful sleep because of fibromyalgia, her complaints might also be magnified and appear to be psychological in nature.

While there is still some controversy regarding fibromyalgia and psychological problems, I have seen that when patients reduce stress in their lives, they also experience a reduction in depression, anxiety, and fatigue, as sleep becomes more restful. Because they feel more in control, the symptoms that were once immobilizing subside and quality of life is realized.

The Mind/Body Interplay

In simplest terms, stress is a response of the body to any demand. It is a biological phenomenon that affects both the central and autonomic nervous systems, as well as the endocrine and immune systems. And it is a key contributing factor to illness, including heart disease, depression, anxiety disorders, asthma and allergy, cancer, and even fibromyalgia.

While there is still some controversy regarding the role of stress in fibromyalgia, there are theories that suggest that it is the annoying daily hassles, not major life stressors, that greatly affect these patients and their symptoms. Especially when coupled with low levels of support from family, friends, co-workers, and even personal physicians, psychological stress may increase the patient's reaction to pain and escalate the chances that pain will occupy her attention. Some theorize that those with fibromyalgia experience higher levels of life stress and lower levels of social support than do healthy individuals.

Evaluate Your Stress Level

How often do you feel stressed? Some patients tell of feeling too much stress during the time when their symptoms flare. On the other hand, many fibromyalgia patients admit that they feel stressed every minute of every day. A recent survey found that 16 percent of those questioned felt stressed "all the time" and could not seem to relax, not even for a minute, while 52 percent of those questioned felt stressed "most of the time."

Every week an estimated 95 million Americans suffer a

stress-related problem and take medication for their aches and pains. There are estimates that as much as 80 percent of all illness is stress-related, and 85 percent of all industrial accidents are linked to personal worker behavior that includes adaptation to stress. In new data from a study done by the Massachusetts Institute of Technology Analysis Group, researchers estimate that depression, which can be triggered by ongoing stress, costs American business $43.7 billion a year— as much as heart disease.

Because stress can show itself through a wide variety of physical changes and emotional responses in fibromyalgia, it is important to identify what causes these feelings. Stress symptoms vary greatly from one person to the next, and learning to identify the ways in which your body and mind show stress is an important step in treating and managing this disease.

SOME EARLY WARNING SIGNS OF STRESS
Anger
Anxiety
Back pain
Body aches and pains
Boredom
Bossiness
Change in bowel or bladder habits
Compulsive eating or gum chewing
Constant worrying
Crying
Dizziness
Dry mouth
Feeling of doom
Forgetfulness
Headaches and other aches
Inability to make decisions

Increased usage of drugs, alcohol, or cigarettes
Indigestion
Lack of creativity
Light-headedness
Loneliness
Loss of sense of humor
Memory loss
Palpitations
Racing heart
Restlessness
Ringing in ears
Sleep problems
Sweaty palms
Teeth grinding
Unhappiness

Not All Stress Is Harmful

Stress can be viewed as positive or negative, and the way we interpret the stress creates differences in our personal responses. In the past decade, research in the field of psychoneuroimmunology (PNI) has shown that life's stressors can produce the same initial physical response of adrenaline rush whether the stress is perceived as positive or negative. For example, you may cringe at the thought of skydiving, while your best friend would push to be first in line. Receiving an award and giving an acceptance speech might be considered exciting for one person, while even the thought of being in the spotlight might make another person visibly ill.

This observation also applies to those with fibromyalgia. I've had some patients who wake up anxious about what lies ahead of them, even when their day does not appear to be stressful. Louise told of how she would lie awake at night and anticipate how horrible she was going to feel the next day. "When the alarm goes off, I feel like crying. I'm tired from lack of sleep, my body aches, and I dread starting a new day," she said.

Yet other patients see each day as an opportunity, no matter what their pain or fatigue threshold is at that particular time. Raymond, a forty-one-year-old tax attorney, was diagnosed with fibromyalgia three years ago, yet he is certainly not waiting for this disease to take over his life. "I've got too much to do," Raymond said. "I've revamped my schedule to rest throughout the day, but other than that, I still do the very activities that I want to. I cannot imagine giving in to the pain and fatigue."

Both good and bad stress can affect fibromyalgia. The roles of perceived stress and psychological factors are controversial in fibromyalgia studies. Many reports show that patients report a heightened awareness of symptoms when facing stress, whether good or bad.

Good stress, or eustress. Positive stress, or *eustress,* still signals the fight-or-flight response as does negative stress, but this adrenaline high usually gives us the energy to enjoy the moment. Positive stressors, such as a promotion or buying a new home, have been linked with increased productivity, happiness, and longevity. Yet for the person with a chronic disease, such as fibromyalgia, these positive events can also be interpreted in a negative manner. As one new grandmother told me, "Just thinking about traveling to take care of my new grandbaby makes me anxious and fatigued."

Bad stress, or distress. Negative stress, or *distress,* also signals adrenaline to rush through your body, but it is this type of stress that puts you into the full-blown stress response and if continuous can lead to loss of productivity, burnout, and health problems, including a higher risk of getting diseases. For people with fibromyalgia, negative stressors, such as losing one's job or the illness of a loved one, can make symptoms that were controlled become active once again.

Stress and Fibromyalgia

The following list will give you an idea of what can add to your stress level each day:

THE STRESS IN YOUR LIFE
Waiting in long lines of traffic
Not being able to relax
Having fear of rejection from family and friends
Not getting recognized for abilities at work or home
Coping with too much noise at home or work
Going shopping and having to make choices
Having an overall dull feeling
Having to attend a party with friends
Not being able to express self
Not getting enough sleep
Meeting with the boss about a raise
Waking up feeling tired each day
Getting too much sleep and still feeling tired
Going out to dinner with family and friends
Overall tired feeling all day long
Annoying people
Being the guest of honor at a party
Misplacing or losing things
Going shopping with friends
Inability to concentrate at work or at home
Fear of confrontation with coworkers or family members
Entertaining friends at home

Inability to get close to coworkers or friends
Problems filling out forms
Preparing for the holidays
Dislike of preparing meals each day
Raising active children
Redecorating the house
Receiving a compliment from the boss
Having concerns about health and fibromyalgia
Vacation with family
Getting the yard work completed
Having no energy to do housework
Not having enough money to make ends meet
Too many medical bills, and the insurance won't cover all of
     them
Having to wait in line anywhere
Having to wait to see a doctor
Having a doctor not believe that the symptoms are real
Sexual problems with mate
Marital problems
Physical reaction to weather changes
Not enough energy to keep up in life
Declining physical abilities

After perusing the list, you may wonder why there are no major stressors listed, such as death of a loved one. If what current research indicates is true, patients with fibromyalgia are more stressed with daily hassles than they are with major life intrusions. In other words, waiting in a line of traffic or wondering how you are going to do your housework with all the pain and fatigue may cause you more apparent stress than a sudden crisis.

However, whatever your problems with fibromyalgia, too much stress does not have to be one of them. You can learn to manage your reaction to stress just as you do other areas of your life.

Melding the Body and Mind

Not only have scientists explored how stress may weaken the immune systems, making us susceptible to diseases, they are also discovering how to meld the body and mind with psychological techniques—techniques that you can easily incorporate into your daily routine to reduce the threat to your immune system and well-being.

The key to reducing the stress that accompanies fibromyalgia lies in recognizing the signs and taking active steps to reduce these before the stress further injures your health and self-esteem. It is not difficult to start the stress-reduction program given in this chapter and incorporate it into your daily lifestyle.

Evaluate Your Commitments

BUDGET YOUR TIME

Do you find that there is never enough time in the day? Setting priorities and budgeting your time each day is the first step in gaining balance in your life, thus eliminating needless stress and anxiety. You can begin to do this by making a list of all of your commitments—family, work, community involvement, friends—and eliminating those commitments that are not absolutely necessary. Especially when you live with chronic pain and fatigue, you must allow for times during the day when you are not at your peak performance. This means not complicating your life with a list of activities and commitments that are just not important.

MAKE "TO DO" LISTS DAILY

Write down tasks that face you each day. As you schedule your day, budget ample time to get your work completed by calculating how long it will take to finish each project—then add on an extra fifteen to thirty minutes, to allow yourself to go at a moderate speed instead of in high gear. This will give you leeway, especially on days when pain and fatigue might hold you back from optimum performance.

If you find that you have more tasks scheduled than time available, rewrite your list and prioritize the projects that *must* be done; put the less important projects or activities at the bottom of the list. These can always wait until another day, or you can delegate them to others. Sharing the load is crucial as you learn to balance your day, doing what your body will let you do without excessive pain and fatigue.

Some people prefer to make their To Do lists each morning, while others find that doing it the night before relieves their minds and enables them to sleep soundly.

SCHEDULE YOUR DAY FOR PEAK EFFICIENCY

For those of you who work, staying employed is obviously a major commitment; but working late into the evening hours or seven days a week is something you can—and must—change.

Some people find that stimulation during late afternoon and evening hours makes it even more difficult to experience restful sleep; if you fall into this category, you may want to exclude evening activities. If mornings are your worst time with pain and fatigue, then plan your day around this and make your main commitments, such as business meetings or shopping, during midday or afternoon.

ACCEPT YOUR LIMITATIONS

When Katrina came to see me, she was at the brink of a divorce from her husband of nineteen years. "This disease has ruined my life. Not only have I lost my health, but my marriage is almost over." Through some intense counseling and a greater understanding of fibromyalgia, Katrina and her husband have worked through their marital problems. But first, she had to accept her limitations. Instead of denying the disease's existence and feeling anger and resentment for its symptoms, Katrina has come to accept it as a new part of her life, realizing that it is not terminal and learning to work around the symptoms to do the very things she enjoys.

Many of the fibromyalgia patients I've treated tell of always trying to achieve the best in whatever they do, and researchers are finding that perfectionism may be an identifying factor for those with this disease. A constant push for perfection can cause undue stress, which results in hazards to mental and physical well-being. Make sure that in all you do, the amount of time you put into the activity or job is well worth the end result. If it isn't, back off and let go of the perfectionistic attitude.

Which of the following perfectionistic beliefs motivate you each day?

- I must achieve my best, no matter how badly I feel.
- I cannot accept anything but perfection in all I do, or I criticize myself harshly.
- No matter how hard I try, I never feel like I've done enough or given enough.
- I would rather work at being perfect than spend pleasurable time with family and friends.

To reduce stress associated with fibromyalgia, you must realize that as a human being you are imperfect, even though you are endeavoring to become something more than you are now. Accepting this tension, you can begin to make some changes in your expectations of yourself. These changes can help you relax so that you can enjoy your life and experience a greater sense of well-being.

IDENTIFY YOUR PERSONAL STRESS REACTION

The initial impact of fibromyalgia on someone is always one of increased reactivity. This means that normally you may be able to handle a large workload, but now that you suffer with symptoms like constant fatigue, general feelings of anxiety or sadness, and muscle aches, any extra stress will put you in reactive gear. When we are in reactive gear, we are driven impulsively by our emotions and how we feel. Not only does reactive gear make us feel vulnerable, it can affect our relationships at home and on the job in a negative manner.

Determine how your body responds to additional stress now that you have been diagnosed with fibromyalgia. What are your stress warning signs as shown on pages 78 and 79? By knowing your own specific stress reactions, you can learn to listen to your body before the stress immobilizes you.

IDENTIFY AND REMOVE STRESS

The main strategy in dealing with stress is to identify and remove or reduce the source. If you react to the stress of being overworked, learn to delegate at your office or at home. If your stress is from overextending yourself with outside commitments, rethink how to modify your priorities and put this plan into action. If your stress stems from the fear of going to bed each night knowing that you are going to toss and turn, try to improve this by using the information in chapter 7 to ensure sounder sleep. If your stress is from facing each day knowing that you may have pain and fatigue, plan ahead the night before. For example, if you set out your clothes and get up thirty minutes earlier, you can move slowly without the necessity of hurrying.

As you seek to minimize stress, ask yourself the following:

- What stressors can I eliminate in my life?
- What stressors can I avoid?

- How can I reduce their intensity or manage them?
- What strategies do I need to use to make these changes?

MAKE JOB-SITE MODIFICATIONS

Fibromyalgia patients who are able to work outside the home tell of experiencing great stress on the job. Some tell of fearing they may be let go as healthier and more qualified workers enter the job force, while others are concerned that they are not able to perform the way they used to. Employers also tell of being concerned with the output of chronically ill patients, citing reduced productivity, increased absenteeism, poor work quality, and increased rates of on-the-job accidents.

To continue to be a productive employee, you need to stay mentally and physically able to handle your job responsibilities. You may need to allow more time during the day to get your responsibilities completed. Elizabeth told of talking with her employer about her illness and working out a plan that would benefit both. "I realized that I became very tired during midday," she said. "At that time, I was of no use to anyone, so with my boss's consent, I mapped out a plan to get my work completed on these bad days by taking a two-hour lunch break to nap, then staying a bit later to finish my reports. It has worked for both of us."

Other job-site modifications might involve taking work home on days when you feel fatigued or working on a Saturday morning so you can take extra long lunch breaks during the week to rest. Whatever you do, avoid procrastination. This may give you a break initially, but when it comes time for the work to be completed, you will feel more stress than ever. It has been said that procrastinators are perfectionists just waiting for that perfect time to do their work. Remember, there is no perfect time! Budget your time, follow your daily To Do lists, and limit your outside commitments on workdays.

Other steps for modifying work stress include:

- Ask for help from coworkers on days when pain and fatigue are overwhelming. Pay them back with your assistance on days when you feel better.
- Take periodic breaks to avoid getting overtired or stressed during busy workdays.
- Listen to music during your workday if you can to help keep stress levels low (see chapter 6 for benefits of music therapy).

Coping with work stress requires that you keep things in perspective. Again, this means that you must seek a balance between self, family, community, and work. This will help you maintain a support network to keep you centered and enable you to have strength to get through the day—even when symptoms flair.

INCREASE COMMUNICATION SKILLS

With a chronic disease like fibromyalgia, communication is the most important tool you have to decrease conflict with family, friends, and coworkers, especially when you feel anger or resentment from having unending pain and fatigue. Preoccupation with your illness causes a tremendous amount of distracting mental activity that can hinder productive communication. If you are feeling overwhelmed by the stress of fibromyalgia, you may find it necessary to have psychological counseling to help you develop appropriate and functional communication strategies to deal with your disease and its effect on your life.

Learn to say "no." Failing to set limits or say no to too many demands will put you in overload and add to your already rising stress level. Try to reach any decision that will involve a physical and mental commitment before you are put on the spot. It is much easier to say no to a persuasive friend when you have thought out the situation beforehand and have checked your calendar. Weigh the alternatives of making a new commitment, and include family members or friends in the discussion. Would another commitment prevent you from getting the rest, exercise, and relaxation you need to feel well? Would it take away from those priorities that are foremost on your list?

The desire to help others is commendable. But if being all things to all people is hindering your healing and making you feel resentful, tired, and depressed, it is time to take a firm stand. Say no—and mean it. You will feel physically and emotionally stronger if you make only those commitments that you can keep without undue stress.

learn to remove yourself emotionally from stressful situations. Sometimes we magnify problems, making them seem far greater than they are. The stress reaction is triggered by our perception. When we imagine something to be a life-and-death situation, our bodies react as if we are in danger, even if no danger exists.

Work at tempering your emotions as problems come up throughout the day. Instead of every crisis being horrible, learn to view life's interruptions as inconvenient but tolerable. You will find that when you see life as something that you can easily handle, it will not overpower you when trouble hits.

KEEP A DAILY JOURNAL

Writing in a journal every day can lend itself to great self-inquiry and allow us to experience a higher plane of consciousness—with enhanced awareness, along with the practice of self-discipline.

With any chronic disease, patients often hide or are even unaware of intense feelings of resentment, anger, and loss. The intense self-inquiry process of keeping a journal can open the pathways to discover these destructive inner feelings and deepest concerns. Some patients can even identify a series of events that are associated with the beginning of fibromyalgia symptoms, offering a possible cause of how and when the symptoms began.

Keeping a journal can also assist you in tracking your muscle pain and fatigue and what the cause may be. For example, you may write in your journal that you are having great pain and feeling exhausted after working in your garden for several days. Months later, you can look back on this date and begin to see a pattern between the increase in your fibromyalgia symptoms and possible lifestyle triggers. Perhaps you find that you haven't slept well in days. Looking back over your journal will enable you to see any emotional or physical problems you may have had that contributed to the sleep problem.

SOAK IN A WARM BATH

Soaking in a warm bath or hot tub, steaming in a sauna, or standing under a warm shower will serve two purposes. First, it will allow you to relax tense muscles, reducing pain and allowing for easier movement (see chapter 3). Second, some studies show that the warm, moist heat may raise levels of endorphins and decrease levels of stress hormones. There may be an added benefit in that health care professionals who specialize in sleep disorders have also found that a warm bath before bedtime may help sleep to be more restful.

ELIMINATE OR REDUCE CAFFEINE INTAKE

Caffeine is one of the few food products that mimics the stress response. While a little caffeine may make you feel less tired on a bad morning when you've tossed and turned all night, too much can add to your already stressed emotional state, causing a short-term rise in blood pressure and increased heart rate and anxiety levels. Too much caffeine can greatly increase nervousness, which is a problem fibromyalgia patients do *not* need.

As you make plans to de-stress your life, try limiting your amount of caffeine intake or better still, eliminate it altogether. Tea and chocolate drinks contain caffeine as well, plus ingredients like theophylline and theobromine, which also can stimulate the heart and central nervous system. Watch that chocolate candy bar you may eat, for it contains caffeine, too. I have found that there is no exact level of caffeine that is okay for everyone, so most patients choose to stop using it altogether.

FOODS HIGH IN CAFFEINE

Coffee, drip	5 oz. (90–115 mg.)
Coffee, perk	5 oz. (60–125 mg.)
Coffee, instant	5 oz. (60–80 mg.)
Coffee, decaf	5 oz. (2–5 mg.)
Tea, 5-min. steep	5 oz. (40–100 mg.)
Tea, 3-min. steep	5 oz. (20–50 mg.)
Hot cocoa	5 oz. (2–10 mg.)
Cola soft drink	12 oz. (45 mg.)
Chocolate bar	2 oz. (30 mg.)

USE MIND / BODY TOOLS FOR RELAXATION

There is evidence that a variety of relaxation therapies, including meditation, prayer, music therapy, deep abdominal breathing, biofeedback, and visualization, are useful in reducing stress and stress-related illness.

When you meditate and experience the relaxation response, your body switches from the pumping "fight or flight" response into a calmer, more peaceful mood. Studies show that when you withdraw from problems and use mind / body tools for relaxation, you can produce alpha and theta waves consistent with serenity and happiness (see chapter 6).

Balance Your Life to Reduce Stress

In short, I know coping with the ongoing stress of fibromyalgia is not easy, but it is an important step in the treatment plan. High levels of stress can add to the wear-and-tear levels on your body and contribute to the pain, fatigue, and depression you already feel. This, in turn, can make it even more difficult to handle other problems that confront you each day.

As you begin to reduce stress in your life, work for an overall lifestyle balance. Make time to do the things you *want* to do, as well as the things you *have* to do. People with chronic diseases are faced with special demands that healthy people do not have. The task of coping with pain and fatigue each day makes it necessary to keep your priorities in order so you have the energy to reach your daily goals.

Remember, no matter what type of disease, all people with pain are stressed. Likewise, all people with fatigue are stressed. When you combine these two major symptoms in a disease like fibromyalgia, it makes it even more difficult to handle everyday issues, much less major life stressors that may arise. While only you can get your life in control, do not feel as if you must do this alone. There are trained professionals ready to guide you and your family in a positive direction that will help you to understand and accept your illness and learn to live a quality life—doing the things you want to do—without restraint.

6

STEP 4:
TRY A COMPLEMENTARY
APPROACH TO RELIEF

Because fibromyalgia has no one set mode of treatment but depends on specific lifestyle changes, many patients have discovered that a complementary approach to healing is very effective in soothing the typical symptoms of pain, depression, and fatigue. Although there have been very few reported studies done on alternative treatments for fibromyalgia, many patients are finding relief. Thelma, a forty-nine-year-old legal secretary and grandmother of two, told of enjoying life too much to allow this chronic illness to bog her down.

At first Thelma was hesitant to tell me of the complementary treatment she had been undergoing, but we finally approached the subject during a recent visit. She told of going to a chiropractor for a weekly body massage and changing her diet dramatically to include vegetarian meals—more soy products and loads of fresh fruits and vegetables—along with supplements of flaxseed oil and antioxidants.

Thelma's dramatic relief from pain was exciting to me, and she was even able to conquer her ongoing sleep problem as she combined the complementary treatment with her medication and prescribed exercise and stress-reduction program.

In my years of medical practice, I have come to welcome it when patients tell me of finding other methods to complement the traditional medical treatment. A recent Harvard

Medical School study noted that one in three adult Americans saw an alternative practitioner in 1990. This number accounted for 425 million visits to unconventional therapists, as opposed to 388 million trips to doctors. A survey taken by the *New England Medical Journal* found that a third of the respondents had used at least one unconventional therapy in the past year and estimated that Americans spent almost $14 billion on those therapies in 1990. Furthermore, nearly all those respondents who use alternative or complementary medicine also see their regular doctors for the same complaint. Interestingly, this same study showed that 72 percent of the people who use alternative treatments do not tell their regular doctors that they are doing so.

My patients tell of using safe forms of alternative or complementary treatment along with their regular medical regime. This treatment may include chiropractic, massage, acupuncture, and dietary supplements, and some find that these add a boost for healing, especially for chronic muscle pain.

The efficacy of many popular complementary forms of treatment has hardly been proven. Therefore, in talking with patients who favor complementary treatments, I discuss the pros and cons of using each, and evaluate the benefit to the disease. It is only after discussing this individually with each patient that I offer my support—if the following two criteria are met:

1. The patient finds that the complementary treatment makes them feel better;
2. The complementary treatment does not hurt the patient in any way.

Let's look at some of the most common forms of complementary treatment.

CHIROPRACTIC

"It took just three visits with my chiropractor until I felt relief from the deep pain in my back and shoulders," said Mac, a thirty-nine-year-old computer salesman. Sarah's story was very similar: "I had no energy at all until I started going to a chiropractor. At first I was skeptical, but after several visits, I began to feel as if my body was working for me instead of against me."

Does chiropractic really work? It all depends on what it is used for. Chiropractic medicine comes closer to traditional Western medicine than the other forms described in this chapter. It is a drug-free approach to health that relies on manipulation of the spine and muscles. Doctors of chiropractic are unique in that instead of treating the symptoms of a patient, they are primarily interested in treating the spinal bones when they lose their normal position and motion from stress, trauma, or other causes.

How does it work? According to doctors of chiropractic, your nervous system controls all functions in your body; every cell in your body is supplied with nervous impulses. Messages must travel from your brain down your spinal cord, then out to nerves to the particular parts of the body, then back to the spinal cord and back up the spinal cord to the brain. The theory is that abnormal positions of the spinal bones may interfere with these messages and oftentimes are the underlying cause of many health problems.

Doctors of chiropractic correct the abnormal positions of the spinal bones with an *adjustment* or *spinal manipulation.* Using his hands or a specially designed instrument, the doctor delivers a brief and accurate thrust to a joint that is fixated, locked up, or not moving properly. Adjustments help return the bones to a more normal position or motion, relieving pain and ill health.

The chiropractic doctor will also recommend a program of

rehabilitation for your spine. This phase of care is analogous to orthodontics. Goals are to stabilize and reduce joint involvement, rehabilitate muscle ligament tissue, and balance nerve impulses, helping you to regain maximum health. Patients who get significant relief from spinal manipulation find that it helps them to continue with their basic treatment plan of heat and exercises and allows them to resume a more normal lifestyle. Additionally, manipulation by a doctor of chiropractic, osteopathy, or other practitioner can be part of a total team approach to treatment with a neurologist, orthopedic surgeon, or rheumatologist to bring about the best total results for that patient.

Many practitioners can do manipulation, including chiropractors and osteopaths. Chiropractic deals primarily with the neuromuscular skeletal system (nerves, muscles, and bones). Osteopathy is a system of medical practice that emphasizes the manipulation of muscles and bones to relieve certain disorders.

THERAPEUTIC TOUCH

Joan, a forty-eight-year-old fibromyalgia patient, said that she gave up her weekly appointment with her hairdresser in exchange for an appointment for *therapeutic touch* (TT) with a physical therapist. Beatrice was a convert, too, saying, "After aching for years with no relief from this fibromyalgia, I found TT so soothing and relaxing, as if the pain is radiated outward by the touch of the therapist's hands." Another patient, Jim, found that the deep pressure he felt on his muscles during massage helped to alleviate the pain in his shoulders and upper back.

When you are very stressed and your muscles are tense, they build up lactic acid. This makes the muscles even more tense, but TT, a holistic philosophy for pain management, can help to relieve this. Studies released by the University of Miami School of Medicine's Touch Research Center found that the benefits of massage include heightened alertness, relief from depression and anxiety, an increase in the number of natural "killer cells" in the immune system, lower levels of the stress hormone cortisol, and reduced difficulty in getting to sleep. Another study reported that patients who received TT for pain-related ailments took fewer narcotics or sedatives for the pain—an important benefit for fibromyalgia patients. Patients have also reported a decreased heart rate and blood pressure and even a reduced skin temperature.

Therapeutic touch affects the body as a whole. This form of drugless therapy has been shown to increase circulation, give relief from musculoskeletal pain, act as a mind / body form of stress release, increase flexibility, and increase mobility.

If you would like to find a qualified, licensed massage therapist, the American Massage Therapy Association provides a national referral service for qualified professional massage therapists.

The therapeutic touch also:

- relieves muscle spasm and tension
- relieves tension-related headaches and headaches associated with fibromyalgia
- strengthens the immune system
- reduces blood pressure
- improves digestion
- creates a calmer mind / body state
- relaxes nervous system and reduces anxiety
- releases endorphins (natural painkillers)
- can increase the levels of serotonin (a natural antidepressant)

ACUPUNCTURE
This ancient form of Chinese medicine has been practiced for more than two thousand five hundred years, yet Western science does not always fully acknowledge its benefit. Acupunc-

ture is becoming more prevalent in the United States and is practiced by doctors who have their main degree in medicine, osteopathy, or chiropractic and who have taken training in the field of acupuncture.

Acupuncture is a form of hyperstimulation for pain relief. There seems to be a close correlation between tender (or trigger) points and acupuncture sites used for pain control. A recent study published in the *British Medical Journal* compared two groups of patients with fibromyalgia. One group was treated with electroacupuncture and the other was given sham treatment during which acupuncture needles were inserted but somewhat less deeply, at a small distance from usually prescribed acupuncture sites, and with a slightly weaker electric current. There was improvement in actively treated patients in terms of duration of morning stiffness, overall pain, sleep quality, and overall assessment of disease compared with baseline. There was no significant improvement in the control group. These results were comparable to those reported for some medical treatments, such as with the antidepressant drug Elavil (amitriptyline) (see pages 48 and 49).

Western medicine research into the subject tells us that acupuncture brings relief through certain reflexes in the body that occur by way of the nervous system. That is to say, by stimulating one portion of the body and using pathways of the nervous system, an effect is obtained in the same or other portion of the body. Additionally, it is believed that acupuncture causes the body to release endorphins, the body's own pain-relieving chemicals.

Acupuncture treatment consists of the placement of fine-gauge sterilized needles at various points selected by the practitioner; for instance, to treat back pain, the practitioner will select some local sites along the spine as well as some distant points on the arms or legs. The needles are usually left in place fifteen to thirty minutes. The doctor may periodically stimulate the needles by manually twisting them to obtain improved results.

Traditional Asian acupuncturists place the needles into specific acupuncture points along the body on lines known as *meridians.* Western doctors utilize the same points, but often also utilize local trigger points—knotted areas in the muscle—that may be responsible for causing the localized or referred pain. Acupuncture may therefore assist those with chronic, deep muscle pain, such as fibromyalgia patients.

Another form of stimulating the acupuncture points once the needle is in place is through hooking up small wires that are connected to very slight electrical currents. This is known as electroacupuncture. There are also ways of applying acupuncture today that do not require needles. Very sophisticated pieces of electronic equipment help the doctor detect the local acupuncture point and treat it with electrical microcurrents. Some patients report good results with this method of acupuncture.

If you want to try acupuncture, keep in mind that you'll need to go through a series of at least eight to ten treatments in order to ascertain whether it will be effective for you. You may not feel any relief, or you may feel extremely long-lasting relief. However, be sure to go to a licensed practitioner who uses disposable needles.

Though acupuncture has very few contraindications and the side effects are minimal, if any, certain disorders such as easy bleeding and local infection may preclude you from receiving acupuncture treatments. You should check with your doctor before trying this form of treatment.

RELAXATION RESPONSE

As we've seen, the daily stress of worrying about fibromyalgia and the limitations that accompany it can create an overload of emotional and mental demands on a person.

The relaxation response, first described by Dr. Herbert Benson more than twenty years ago, is one of the most studied methods to reduce stress. Learning to induce the relaxation response at will can offer a real potential to reduce physical strain and emotional, negative thoughts—and increase your ability to self-manage stress.

Learn to Relax

Relaxation may be easy for some, but most people, even when they think they are relaxing, are not aware of the enormous muscle tension running throughout the body. By allowing time in your daily schedule to practice the suggested mind / body therapy and alternative treatment in this chapter, you can begin to get in touch with this muscle tension and learn how to end it—permanently.

I know how difficult it is to structure time for relaxation each day. Just the thought of making time to take a leisurely walk actually makes some people even more stressed! But I also know that if you will plan for as little as ten to twenty minutes, twice a day, to practice these mind / body techniques, you will learn to relax, even under the most stressful situations. As you do this, blood flow to the brain will increase, enabling brain waves to shift from an alert, beta, rhythm to a relaxed, alpha, rhythm.

Your body will soon learn to get into a relaxation mode, and you can target the sympathetic nervous system. This, in turn, will result in a more relaxed feeling and help to quiet the anxiety often felt by fibromyalgia patients. It will also help to induce a more restful stage 4 sleep. Some studies of late have revealed that not only is relaxation important for getting in touch with tension, but after a period of relaxation, people feel more joyful, creative, optimistic, and loving.

No matter how severe your fibromyalgia symptoms are,

perhaps the most important element for winning with mind / body interplay is believing that it will work. This approach to wellness requires your active participation and total involvement in health and healing as you learn and perform the various modes of therapy. It is one important part of your treatment program that depends totally on you for success.

If you find it hard to relax on your own or if you are interested in learning more about an individual approach for relaxation and stress management, it would be a good idea to see a clinical psychologist who specializes in working with these problems. Whether you use the techniques discussed in this book or choose formal training by a professional, learning to relax effectively can help control the emotional problems involved with fibromyalgia, increase your positive thinking, and lessen the impact of this disease on your overall lifestyle.

MUSIC THERAPY

Music therapy has proven to be an effective nonpharmacologic approach to assist in reducing fear, anxiety, stress, or grief in chronically ill patients. It is just beginning to make its mark as a way to treat pain and the stress that accompanies it, yet many are already reporting it to be the best way to lower stress. Some researchers have found that in studies with chronic pain patients, the use of music can cause patients to have a higher tolerance of pain.

Music therapy may sound too easy to work, but many of the sensations arising from music and pain are processed in the same areas of the brain. These areas are also responsible for coordinating our emotional responses. Thus, by focusing on and responding to music, we can block the body's response to pain. With this relaxation, we can decrease muscle tension and increase endorphin levels. While the level of pain does not change, having less tension and anxiety can make the pain tolerable.

For de-stressing with fibromyalgia and for pain reduction, it is helpful to try music therapy in combination with another mind / body technique, such as guided imagery (visualization), deep abdominal breathing, or progressive muscle relaxation, as discussed in the following pages. This will enhance the inner peace you are experiencing.

If you employ music therapy as part of your treatment program, make sure that the pace of the music you choose is slightly slower than your heart rate, or approximately 60 beats a minute. This rhythm encourages your heart rate to slow down; some studies of late have shown that this will also lower blood pressure. The works of Vivaldi and Chopin fit into this category, or you might try New Age music by artists like George Winston.

DEEP ABDOMINAL BREATHING

Breathing can measure and alter your psychological state, making a stressful moment accelerate or diminish in intensity. Think about how your respiration quickens when you are fearful or in great pain and how taking a deep, slow breath can have a calming effect, reducing both stress and levels of muscle pain.

But how often we take breathing for granted! This is one of the few activities of the body that we can consciously control. As you learn how to do deep abdominal breathing, you will gain control over a basic physiological function, helping to decrease the release of stress hormones and slow down your heart rate during stressful moments. Also, by adding oxygen to the blood, you can actually cause your body to release endorphins, those hormones that give a greater sense of well-being and contentment.

Lie on your back in a quiet room with no distractions. If necessary, take the phone off the hook so you are truly alone. Place your hands on your abdomen and take a slow, deliberate deep breath in through your nostrils. If your hands are rising, your abdomen is expanding and you are breathing correctly. If your hands do not rise, yet you see your chest rising, you are breathing incorrectly.

Inhale to a count of five, pause for three seconds, then exhale to a count of five. Start with ten repetitions of this exercise, then increase to twenty-five, twice daily. Use this exercise any time you feel anxious or stressed. Some of my patients find it extremely helpful when they are experiencing great pain. As one patient, Laura, said, "When I have severe muscle pain, I use my breathing to go with the pain. Somehow, this takes my mind off the pain and lessens its severity."

PROGRESSIVE MUSCLE RELAXATION

Progressive muscle relaxation involves contracting and relaxing all the different muscle groups in the body, beginning with the head and neck and progressing down to the arms, chest, back, stomach, pelvis, legs, and feet. To do this exercise, you focus on each set of muscles, tense these muscles to the count of ten, then release to the count of ten. Go slowly as you progress throughout your entire body, taking as long as you can. Get in touch with each part and feel the tension you are experiencing. Notice how it feels to be tension-free as you release the muscle.

Studies show that when you can create a strong mental image using this type of relaxation technique, you actually feel "removed" from cumbersome stress and negative emotions. This mindfulness, or focusing all attention on what you feel from moment to moment, can also help you move beyond destructive habits as you become centered in a world of health and inner healing.

You can do this exercise with or without music, and it is important to perform it with deep abdominal breathing. Focusing on your breathing, breathe in while tensing the muscles, and exhale while relaxing them.

GUIDED IMAGERY TECHNIQUES

According to scientific tests, the mind cannot distinguish between fears, fantasies, and reality as we understand it. Therefore, another effective mind / body technique for healing is guided imagery (also called visualization). This involves mentally seeing pictures of relaxing situations, such as a beach at sunset, a flowing mountain waterfall, or a brilliant mountain sunrise.

Guided imagery is a technique that all people have the potential to master. Some of us are naturally better at imagining than others, but we can all learn to visualize effectively if we practice. Much like learning to play the piano or tennis, becoming skilled at guided imagery involves time, patience, and practice. This is a skill that cannot be rushed or hurried.

The power of your imagination is important in guided imagery as you use sights, sounds, feelings, and smell to create a desired state in your mind. Used in combination with deep breathing, it produces long-term stress reduction. This technique has been used to improve the surveillance function of the immune system. Through guided imagery, you will reduce your anxiety level during stressful times and lower your heart rate and blood pressure. As you continuously visualize a positive healing image, you may significantly contribute to your own well-being.

If you have trouble imagining scenes and images, listen to sounds of waves or thunderstorms to trigger images of natural settings. These recordings can be purchased at any music store. Or take photographs of peaceful, serene scenes and keep these with you. Pull out your visualization cards when you feel your body tensing and you need to imagine being somewhere else where life is kinder and less threatening.

BIOFEEDBACK

Biofeedback training has been shown to bring about improvement in the number of tender points and morning stiffness in some fibromyalgia patients. Biofeedback is based on the idea that when people are given information about their body's internal processes, they can use this information to learn to control those processes.

Many studies have affirmed the use of biofeedback as a mind / body approach in fibromyalgia patients. In one study, fifteen fibromyalgia patients who had a poor response to medication treatment were trained with biofeedback. After a fifteen-session biofeedback program, these patients improved in tender-point count, pain rating, and morning stiffness.

When taught by a qualified licensed psychologist, the patient can control responses of the body using biofeedback, resulting in less pain and stress. Other physiological responses, such as heart rate, sweat production, hand temperature, or breathing patterns may also be monitored and provide more information for the patient and psychologist.

Biofeedback requires you to be connected to a machine that informs you and your therapist when you are physically relaxing your body. With sensors placed over specific muscle sites, the therapist can read the tension in your muscles, the amount of sweat you are producing, or the temperature of your finger. Any one or all of these readings can let the trained biofeedback therapist know if you are learning to relax.

The ultimate goal of biofeedback is to use this skill when you are facing real stressors, away from the therapist's office. If learned successfully, biofeedback can help you control your heart rate, blood pressure, and muscle tension. Some therapists recommend tapes that can be listened to at home to practice relaxation techniques.

HYPNOSIS

Hypnosis is another way to control the pain and stress that accompany fibromyalgia and has been endorsed by the American Psychiatric Association and the American Psychological Association. Although hypnosis comes from the Greek word meaning "sleep," it is really an intense state of focused concentration.

In one controlled trial, hypnotherapy patients reported less pain, less fatigue on awakening, and better sleep patterns than patients receiving physical therapy alone.

While hypnosis is not a new method of treatment, it is now being used in new ways to improve the quality of life of chronic pain patients. During a hypnosis session, suggestions are made to the patient that allow her to decrease the intensity of the pain, to move the pain to another area, or to try to build a feeling of separation from the pain.

While this may sound too easy to work, hypnosis has been used successfully to help chronic pain in limited studies. I recommend that it be used to supplement other methods of pain control, such as exercises and medications.

If done correctly, this type of mind / body therapy can produce a feeling of calm and improve a patient's confidence in handling the symptoms of fibromyalgia. Because hypnosis is not meant for everyone and may not work with every person, you should seek a qualified clinical psychologist or psychiatrist to help you decide if hypnosis would be helpful and safe for you.

AROMATHERAPY

At this time, research is being conducted on aromas or scents and how they may alter one's moods and thoughts. Some studies have been done on inhalation of scents, yet *aromatherapy* extends far beyond this to include the use of certain oils. Each oil is suggested to have a specific healing power, whether to reduce stress, fight infection, increase energy, or serve as an aphrodisiac. For example, studies have been done on the odor of spiced apples, and conclusions have been drawn that this scent produces feelings of relaxation. Other scents, such as lemon, make people more alert. Some research has found chamomile oil to be anti-inflammatory and clove oil to be antimicrobial.

While it has been found that odors can change brain wave states, how do scientists explain the connection between odor and mood? Exactly how the scent-mood link works remains a mystery. Researchers do know that when aromatic molecules drift into the nose, they lock on to receptors there and create electrical impulses that travel up the olfactory nerves to the brain. One destination is the limbic system, where emotions and memory are processed. There is widespread agreement that these aromas help to increase the quality of sensory input for patients, thus reducing levels of stress. For example, lavender has been found to increase alpha wave activity in the back of the brain, a sign of relaxation.

So does aromatherapy really work? While there have been no controlled studies to date, claims rest on patients who say they have been healed or at least made to feel better with aromatherapy. Therefore, the answer to whether scents can change one's mood and reduce stress may actually depend upon the individual.

Sometimes fragrant oils are used in conjunction with therapeutic touch to ease the tension on the skin surface. These oils not only feel soothing to the touch, but also have scents that can evoke tranquility.

There is a national professional organization, the National Association for Holistic Aromatherapy, along with a host of treatment centers across the nation specializing in this mind / body approach to healing and pain relief.

Prayer and Meditation

Many of my patients tell of using prayer and meditation to give comfort during times of pain. One young mother told of how prayer helped control her pain level so she could get through her daily activities. Another woman practices meditation daily for more than an hour each time. She said that this helps her to focus on her healing and frees her from the bondage of the disease.

Both of these spiritual disciplines allow your thoughts to take a break from daily analytical routines and give support to the spiritual dimension of life. When you pray or meditate, your body moves into a calmer, more peaceful state. Studies show that both prayer and meditation produce alpha and theta waves consistent with serenity and happiness. Prayer and meditation provide nourishment for your soul, satiate that inner spiritual hunger, and help you develop your ability to pay attention to all areas of life without distraction.

Can prayer and meditation help control the symptoms of fibromyalgia? Again, although there is no proof that these mind / body tools cause healing, there are more and more studies showing that those who find strength and comfort in their religion have greater survival rates from serious disease.

FOCUS ON NATURE

Our bodies, minds, and spirits need the opportunity to celebrate our existence on this planet, to find meaning in nature. Try to take time-outs each day to focus on nature and natural settings so that your mind does not dwell on worries about your health.

These time-outs can be as uncomplicated as

- pausing to reflect on a brilliant sunrise
- having a cup of herbal tea midafternoon while watching birds feed out-of-doors

- sitting at the edge of the ocean, watching the waves crash upon the shore
- staring at an aquarium of tropical fish
- meditating as you gaze at a peaceful painting

TAI CHI

The Arthritis Foundation reports that tai chi may be a perfect exercise for arthritis sufferers. Tai chi is a Chinese martial art that is used for coping with tension and stress. It can offer tremendous benefits to fibromyalgia sufferers, as it emphasizes complete relaxation and passive concentration without risk of injury. Some have even said that it is like meditation in motion, with dramatic, flowing movements instead of forceful actions. The ultimate goal of tai chi is to bring the principles of yin and yang into natural harmony. For those who find exercise painful, tai chi may enable you to slowly move your body in a full range of motion, building strength while also receiving the benefit of stress reduction.

Studies show that using tai chi for as little as three months can lower blood pressure to normal levels and give improved blood circulation and increased energy. And people who enjoy this form of moving meditation regularly tell of its making them aware of every part of their body.

There are books on tai chi, as well as videos that you can purchase and use in the privacy of your home.

Homeopathic Medicine

Homeopathy is a therapeutic system of medicine that started in the late eighteenth century. It is based on the principle of "like cures like symptom," which means that remedies that would cause a potential problem in large doses will actually encourage the body to heal more rapidly if given in small doses. Practitioners use small diluted formulas of plant, mineral, and animal substances to treat various ailments, hoping to stimulate the body's reaction to throw off the offender. Though homeopathic remedy sales are rapidly growing by 25 percent a year according to the National Center for Homeopathy in Alexandria, Virginia, this type of alternative medical treatment has always received great scrutiny by the traditional medical community. If you seek advice from a homeopathic practitioner, be sure this person is a medical doctor, and check with your own physician before taking an unknown substance that promises great cures.

HERBAL THERAPY
Herbal and other plant-derived remedies have been estimated by the World Health Organization (WHO) to be the most frequently used therapies worldwide. Although precise levels of use in the United States are unknown, herbal products accounted for sales of more than $1.6 billion in 1994, and constitute the fastest-growing category in drugstores.

Pharmaceutical companies are very interested in herbal therapy, and reports are that more than 25 percent of all prescription drugs are derived from these wild medicinals, including the flowers, leaves, bark, berries, and roots of plants. While there are a few herbs that are dangerous and should never be ingested or put on your skin, most herbs are safe.

Keep in mind if you do choose to do herbal therapy that some therapeutic agents derived from plants include pure chemical entities available as prescription drugs (e.g., morphine). Plant-derived remedies can contain chemicals with potent pharmacologic toxicologic properties.

The problem with trying to purchase herbs that are guaranteed safe is that there is no proof that herbal therapies work, other than word-of-mouth from consumers. In order to get FDA approval, the company marketing a drug must prove that it is safe and effective. Since plants cannot be patented, most companies call herbal medicine "foods" and market them in this way.

Herbal remedies have been used for generations and can be put in tea, soup, or taken in other forms. Certain remedies, such as alfalfa or chamomile, are more popular in some areas of this country than in others. While some herbal therapies have not been shown to have a specific benefit for arthritis symptoms, some patients have used the following with good results for helping to obtain more restful sleep or for more energy.

BLACKCURRANT SEED OIL. Although the studies are just now taking place on herbal therapies with various types of arthritis, blackcurrant seed oil has been found in some studies to be helpful in reducing the signs and symptoms of disease activity in patients with rheumatoid arthritis.

Blackcurrant seed oil is rich in inerrant seed oil gammalinolenic acid (GLA) and alphalinolenic acid (ALA). Both GLA and eicosapentaenoic acid (EPA), which derives from ALA, suppress inflammation and joint tissue injury in animal models. In one particular study, patients with rheumatoid arthritis given a placebo showed no change in the disease, while patients who took blackcurrant seed oil (BCSO) showed improvement. How this herb relates to fibromyalgia is still unknown.

BOSWELLIA. Boswellia acids come from a large tree in India and have been demonstrated to have anti-inflammatory effects in animal studies. It has traditionally been used for treatment of osteoarthritis, although some studies have found good results in rheumatoid treatment. No side effects from boswellia have been reported.

CHAMOMILE. This is one of the most common herbs and can be found in most supermarkets as an herbal tea. Chamomile has been used for years to treat nervousness, upset stomach, and menstrual cramps. Its history as a tranquilizer is scientifically based, as this herb depresses the central nervous system. It may also aid in boosting immune power. If you have allergies, be cautious with chamomile, as it contains pollen.

FEVERFEW. This herb grows wild in Europe and has been used to treat arthritis and chronic headaches. Those who use feverfew claim that it is most effective when used to prevent pain and swelling instead of taking it after these symptoms have occurred. Researchers have reported that it may inhibit inflammation and act similarly to aspirin. Those with migraine headaches may be particularly interested in this herb.

Anyone with a clotting disorder should consult their physician before taking feverfew, as it could create a health hazard.

GINSENG. Ginseng has been used for centuries to increase energy and relieve stress. There are various types of ginseng, including Chinese and American varieties; the Siberian ginseng, however, is a different type of plant. Some claim that ginseng can stimulate special enzymes that promote elimination of toxic foreign substances, as well as increase the immune response by stimulating the number of antibodies in the body. Ginseng has also been reported to stimulate memory, counteract fatigue, and soothe damage caused by stress.

If you try ginseng, be cautious, because too much can cause nervousness and insomnia.

KELP. Proponents of using kelp claim that it provides energy and endurance, helps relieve nervous tension, and promotes circulation to the brain. Kelp is said to contain almost every mineral needed. Some fibromyalgia patients claim that kelp helps to increase their energy level, while others say that it has no effect at all.

MEADOWSWEET. This is the herb from which salicylic acid was first obtained and has been used for a long time to treat rheumatism and arthritis. It is grown in the United States and Canada. Because of the aspirinlike quality, be cautious taking it if you have a blood disorder or are on any anti-inflammatory medication, such as an NSAID.

PASSIONFLOWER. This herb, also known as apricot vine or water lemon, is used frequently as a mild tranquilizer and may also be helpful for easing insomnia, stress, and anxiety.

PINE BARK. This is an ancient remedy for arthritis and rheumatism used in Europe, East Asia, and China. The essential oil containing pinene is taken from the bark and needles. Pinene is said to stimulate circulation and help reduce inflammation. Another compound found in pine bark is pycnogenol, which is said to boost the action of serotonin. The essential oils from pine bark are used to soothe sore muscles, and tablets of pycnogenol are used to battle the pain of arthritis. This herb does have drawbacks, and in some chronic conditions, such as lupus, it has been found to worsen the illness.

SPIRULINA. Spirulina is one of the few plant sources of vitamin B_{12} and provides high concentrations of chelated minerals, pigmentations, rhamnose sugars, trace elements, and enzymes. Research claims that spirulina is valuable in weight control and in treating allergies, anemia, and other medical conditions.

VALERIAN ROOT. This is a well-known natural remedy for stress and nervousness and can be found in health food stores. The herb contains compounds that have a sedative effect and has been shown to help in treating insomnia. Because the flavor is rather pungent, you may want to add this to a favorite flavored herbal tea, or you can purchase it in pill form. If you are already taking antidepressants, you should stay away from valerian.

TAKE A CAUTIOUS APPROACH TO HERBAL THERAPY

If you want to try herbal therapy, it is important to consult with your physician. Many times you may pick up something at the grocery or health food store because of an advertised "quick cure" for pain and stiffness, but when it comes to self-medicating with herbs, my response is let the buyer beware. Always know what you are putting in your body and on your skin. Because herbal therapies are not approved or regulated by the FDA, they may be combined with other ingredients that could actually make your condition worse. In other words, while most might help your symptoms, others can be deadly.

Be open-minded as you consider alternative treatments for fibromyalgia. You don't want to miss a chance for good relief, but you also don't want to take unnecessary risks.

When patients come to me with a new remedy that is an alternative treatment, I ask them to consider the following:

- Is it approved by the U.S. Food and Drug Administration (FDA)?
- Does it have any known side effects?
- What is the expertise of the person administering the remedy?
- What has happened to similar treatments over the years?
- Will your health insurance company reimburse you?

Become your own expert. Beware of any treatment that promises quick and easy relief or cure. If it sounds too good to be true, it probably is. You can receive more information on alternative treatments from the Arthritis Foundation or Fibromyalgia Association listed on page 153.

It is important to know when a substance may be dangerous to your health, and you should use caution with any substance taken internally. For example, rattlesnake meat is a common remedy in some areas for many illnesses, including arthritis and back pain. But some forms of capsules containing rattlesnake meat have been shown to cause serious illness.

If an alternative treatment is proven harmless and won't delay proper medical evaluation and treatment, then it is acceptable to try. If you have questions about a new treatment, talk to your doctor and make sure it is safe to use. This will allow you to take advantage of newer treatments but avoid those that may cause more harm than relief.

It is my experience that once patients have the diagnosis of fibromyalgia and learn to live with it, they become the experts on their disease; those who tell of feeling more energy and less pain have learned how to make lifestyle changes and use alternative and medical treatments in a complementary manner—in a way that enhances both health and well-being.

7

STEP 5: END SLEEPLESS NIGHTS

Sleep deprivation was written all across Christina's face. Until she started treatment for fibromyalgia two years ago, this forty-seven-year-old woman lived for months with dark circles under her eyes from lack of restful sleep. Christina made it a point to be in bed by nine o'clock each night but then tossed and turned until sunrise and always felt too tired to go to work the next day.

Like Christina, the majority of fibromyalgia patients are fatigued, even after sleeping for ten hours at night. One woman said, "I go to bed tired and feel tired all night. I awaken tired, then I feel tired the next day."

Patients complain that no matter how long they sleep, it is never restful. Their sleep may be interrupted by frequent awakening, i.e., becoming awake enough that they remember these times the next day. Even more common are awakenings that are not enough to remember but that definitely break up their deep sleep. Most patients tell of waking up day after day feeling exhausted. They feel more tired in the morning, and many have great difficulty in concentrating during the day, just as in other situations where sleep is disrupted.

Because obtaining restful sleep is a crucial problem with this disease, it is helpful to understand the characteristics of normal sleep and how this differs from the sleep experienced by fibromyalgia patients.

Understanding the Stages of Sleep

Studies have demonstrated that we have a built-in cycle of sleep-wake times along with many other cyclic variations in bodily functions, such as glandular secretions, body temperature, heart rate, blood pressure, and bronchial function. These intrinsic cycles are controlled by a group of nerve cells called a circadian pacemaker. This pacemaker is closely related to parts of the retina (in the back of the eye) and the hypothalamus in the brain.

The circadian cycle is actually twenty-five hours long. Since the cycle is longer than the twenty-four-hour day, some factor must serve to synchronize the body's pacemaker with the external clock time. These are cues from the environment called *zeitgebers* (from German, meaning "time-givers"). The most important and powerful one is light. The hormone most closely linked to the circadian system is melatonin, which is made by the pineal gland in another part of the brain. Melatonin has been shown to synchronize the sleep-wake cycle to twenty-four hours in some blind subjects who were otherwise unable to live on a twenty-four-hour day and is discussed on page 53.

In adults, sleep is made up of distinct types or stages with specific characteristics defined by brain waves, eye movements, and muscle tension. The two broad categories of sleep include rapid eye movement sleep (REM) and nonrapid eye movement sleep (NREM). During REM sleep, there are small, variable-speed brain waves, rapid eye movements like those of eyes-open wakefulness, and absent muscle tension. It is during REM sleep that we have almost all of our dreams. (Arousals from this stage of sleep are usually associated with recall of vivid imagery.) In NREM sleep, there are four different stages—1, 2, 3, and 4—characterized by different combinations of brain waves, eye movements, and reduced but not absent muscle tension. In fibromyalgia, stages 3 and 4 NREM sleep are of most importance. These stages are defined by relatively large, slow brain waves (delta waves), absent eye movements, and reduced muscle tension. Other names for these stages are "slow-wave sleep" or "delta sleep."

About sixty years ago, it was recognized that sleep intensity is reflected by the amount of delta sleep. The depth of sleep is correlated with this stage, and it is from delta sleep that arousal is most difficult. Interestingly, growth hormone secretion is highest during delta sleep. Some researchers suggest this is important for growth and repair of body tissue.

The stages of sleep can be contrasted with the state of wakefulness. The wake state is associated with small, variable, but mostly rapid (seven to eleven cycles per second) brain waves called alpha waves. There are quick, alert eye movements along with variable, generally high tension in the muscles.

The stages of sleep are distributed through the normal sleep period in a particular pattern. Sleep onset usually is within five to twenty minutes of going to bed. After the start of sleep, there is a cycling through stages 1 to 4 approximately every forty-five to ninety minutes with REM sleep punctuating each cycle at about sixty- to ninety-minute intervals. Delta sleep occurs mostly in the first third of the night and makes up about 10 to 20 percent of total nocturnal sleep in normal young adults, while REM sleep takes place predominantly during the last third of the night's sleep.

The percentage of delta sleep is affected by age, amount of prior sleep, and various diseases. Delta sleep decreases with age and may be absent in healthy, elderly males. Sleep deprivation increases the rapidity of the onset of delta sleep and its portion of total sleep time.

Young children have particularly large proportions of delta sleep, which increases if they are sleep-deprived. This explains why it is frequently difficult to awaken children. Elderly people have smaller proportions of delta sleep, which is why they are easily aroused by environmental noise. Medical problems, such as obstructive sleep apnea, periodic leg movements during sleep, and fibromyalgia may affect quantity and quality of delta sleep. This in turn probably accounts in some measure for the feeling of fatigue experienced by people suffering from these maladies.

Fibromyalgia and Sleep

About twenty years ago, researchers in Toronto discovered that patients with fibromyalgia had NREM stages of sleep "contaminated" by an intercurrent alpha rhythm (like that of wakefulness). But whether the sleep disturbance caused the fibromyalgia symptoms or was secondary to the disease itself could not be determined.

This group of investigators went on to show that healthy subjects selectively deprived of delta sleep by being exposed to noise developed periods of delta sleep mixed with alpha waves. Interestingly, when deprived of delta sleep these people experienced some musculoskeletal discomfort and mood symptoms similar to those of the patients with fibromyalgia. These data suggested that the stage 4 sleep disturbance caused the appearance of the achiness or pain and mood symptoms.

However, it was felt that the effect of delta sleep disturbance on symptoms might be determined by examining the physical and psychological characteristics of the healthy subjects. Their subjects were younger than the patient population with fibromyalgia and free from illnesses and psychological problems, but they were not particularly physically fit. Yet they had the symptoms of fibromyalgia when put through the sleep-deprivation process. Their relatively sedentary lifestyle may have been significant, because most reports have pointed to the positive influence of exercise on delta sleep.

Sleep disturbances can be triggered in patients by physical or emotional trauma or by a metabolic or other medical problem. Poor sleep can lead to fatigue with resultant diminished exercise causing worsened physical fitness and the establishment of a vicious cycle of inactivity and sleep disturbance with physical and mood-related symptoms (see the Cycle of Inactivity on page 61). These problems could help lead to the development of fibromyalgia.

ACCURATE DIAGNOSIS IS ESSENTIAL FOR PROPER THERAPY

Many of the symptoms that fibromyalgia patients experience are shared by those with other sleep disorders. For example, some patients with obstructive sleep apnea, intermittent blockages of the upper airway at the back of the tongue, which occurs in 2 percent of women and 4 percent of men who are thirty to sixty years old, also complain of unrefreshing sleep and "hurting all over" upon arising in the morning. They also have a history of snoring and other symptoms, including morning headaches, dry mouth, and an increased tendency to doze off during the day. Some patients with sleep apnea have high blood pressure.

If your doctor suspects that your sleep disorder may have a different cause, he may recommend that you have a sleep study. Sleep studies, called *polysomnography*, which include an *electroencephalogram* (EEG), which measures the electrical activity of the brain, as well as the monitoring of oxygen levels, movements of chest wall and abdomen, and nasal and oral airflow. A sleep study may show apnea (periods without breathing), manifested by absent airflow at nose and mouth in conjunction with ongoing respiratory muscle efforts shown by movement of chest wall and abdomen. An apnea may cause decreases in blood oxygen levels. Sleep is often interrupted at the end of the apnea by awakening.

This breaking up of continuous sleep is a major cause of daytime fatigue and sleepiness. Periodic leg movements during sleep, also known as nocturnal myoclonus, may also be associated with alpha intrusions and are a common cause of sleep interruptions. These sleep disorders require specific therapy.

It should be noted that certain drug therapy for fibromyalgia may worsen obstructive sleep apnea and actually exacerbate the patient's symptoms of fatigue and restless sleep.

The Problem of Insomnia

Because patients with fibromyalgia have a specific type of insomnia, a disorder of initiating and / or maintaining sleep, it is important to apply certain treatment measures. Not only is attention to sleep hygiene important, but such stimulants as caffeine and nicotine must be avoided near bedtime. Regular daily exercise, including stretching and aerobic activity, is a form of treatment that can help to consolidate sleep and to alleviate other symptoms. Biofeedback and relaxation techniques, as discussed in chapter 6, are useful in overcoming problems of initiating sleep.

High levels of arousal associated with racing thoughts, worrying, or rumination may also delay sleep onset. Meditation or guided imagery (see chapter 6) can be used to help the patient relax while focusing thoughts on a neutral or enjoyable target.

Nutritional and Hormonal Therapy for Sleep Disorders

About forty years ago, pharmacological studies suggested that the hormone serotonin may have a role in sleep induction. Later on, experiments in animals showed that destruction of the parts of the brain that housed serotonin-containing nerve cells could produce total insomnia. Partial damage to these areas of the brain caused variable decreases in sleep. The percentage of destruction of these particular nerve cells was correlated with the amount of slow-wave sleep.

It turns out that a nutrient, an amino acid called tryptophan, is a precursor in the synthesis of serotonin in the brain. Since tryptophan is present in milk—and warm milk seems to help some individuals fall asleep—this amino acid became a popular item at health food stores as the home remedy for insomnia. However, some patients who ingested tryptophan as a dietary supplement developed a syndrome with features of a disease called scleroderma, which included skin tightening, pain in joints, muscle aches, and weakness. These patients also developed anxiety, depression, and difficulty learning. Some patients actually died. It was later thought that the deaths were due to a contaminant of tryptophan in the substance they took.

It needs to be pointed out that not everyone who took the drug experienced side effects. By the same token, not everyone experienced relief of insomnia. Tryptophan, needless to say, fell out of favor as a nutritional supplement and treatment for insomnia and was pulled off the shelves. As discussed in chapter 8, foods rich in carbohydrates can also boost serotonin levels in the brain, helping to induce feelings of sleepiness and relaxation.

Tips to Encourage Sleep

Establishing better sleep hygiene is vital in managing the symptoms of fibromyalgia. In our clinic, patients have experienced great success with the following suggestions:

Sleep only as much as needed to feel refreshed and healthy the following day, not more. Curtailing the time in bed seems to solidify sleep; excessively long times in bed seem related to fragmented and shallow sleep.

A regular arousal time in the morning strengthens circadian cycling and leads to regular times of sleep onset.

A steady daily amount of exercise probably deepens sleep; occasional exercise, however, does not necessarily improve sleep the following night.

Occasional loud noises (e.g., aircraft flyovers) disturb sleep even in people who are not awakened and cannot remember them in the morning. Sound-attenuated bedrooms may help those who must sleep close to noise.

Although excessively warm rooms disturb sleep, there is no evidence that an excessively cold room solidifies sleep.

Hunger may disturb sleep; a light carbohydrate snack before bedtime may help you avoid sleep disturbances.

Caffeine in the evening disturbs sleep, even in those who feel it does not.

Alcohol may help tense people fall asleep more easily, but ensuing sleep is then fragmented.

People who awake feeling angry and frustrated because they cannot sleep should not keep trying, but should turn on the light and do something different. You might have a light snack high in carbohydrates, read a book, or watch a television show in another room.

The chronic use of tobacco disturbs sleep.

Another procedure we use to help patients overcome conditioned insomnia is stimulus-control behavior therapy. The goal is to reassociate the bedroom stimuli with sleep rather than with frustration and arousal. To achieve this, patients are told that they are "misusing" their bed if they lie in it awake and frustrated. Richard Bootzin, the behavior therapist who initiated this approach, recommends the following rules:

Go to bed only when sleepy.

Use the bed only for sleeping; do not read, watch television, or eat in bed.

If unable to sleep, get up and move to another room. Stay up until you are really sleepy, then return to bed. If sleep still does not come easily, get out of bed again. The goal is to associate bed with falling asleep quickly.

Set the alarm and get up at the same time each morning, regardless of how much you slept during the night. This helps the body acquire a constant sleep-wake rhythm.

Do not nap during the day.

If the above rules are followed, patients will usually sleep little during the first night. By the second or third night, patients are so tired that they fall asleep on the first or second attempt. Sleep patterns then fluctuate for a few weeks, but gradually the bedroom surroundings again become associated with sleep. However, most patients need a lot of encouragement during this difficult reconditioning period.

Precise diagnosis is essential to establish the existence of fibromyalgia and to distinguish this disease from other sleep disorders. Once the diagnosis is made, a multifaceted approach is then required to ensure restful and healing sleep and may require some combination of supportive psychotherapy, biofeedback-relaxation techniques, physical fitness training, antidepressants, or some other medicine as discussed in chapter 3, along with careful medical supervision by a physician.

8

STEP 6:
FOLLOW THE NUTRITIONAL
PLAN FOR HEALING

While there are no specific "magic" foods that are proven to cure fibromyalgia, research has shown that there are some positive nutritional measures you can take to heal your body. Being at the proper weight and eating healthful foods, including those that are low in fat and high in immunity-boosting antioxidants and phytochemicals, work together to help maximize energy and alertness, while possibly minimizing the constant fatigue and lethargy that accompany this syndrome.

To be healthy and feel good become increasingly more complicated with chronic diseases like fibromyalgia. Good health is more about the precise balance of a sound body, mind, and spirit than just the absence of disease. There are unique links among the brain, the hormone system, and the immune system. Within this balance, these links make feeling our best a total experience—physical, mental, and emotional. Taking charge of the areas of your health that you *can* control helps to optimize how you feel even in the midst of the aches and fatigue of fibromyalgia.

Taking Control of Your Disease

Eating for wellness is one of the treatment areas that you do have control over. Knowing that you are doing all you can to eat healthily can give you a sense of power to sustain your physical needs and help you cope with the stresses of everyday life and fibromyalgia.

The food choices you make can affect your weight; obesity is a significant public health problem in the United States, as well as in other developed nations. Studies are now being conducted to see if obesity contributes to an impaired immune system. If this is the case, then it is even more necessary that everyone takes control of his or her weight and nutrition.

Nutrients Support Repair of the Body

Nutrients are special compounds found in foods that support the body's repair, growth, and wellness. They include vitamins, minerals, amino acids, essential fatty acids, and water, and the calorie sources of carbohydrate, protein, and fat. Some nutrients can be made by the body (nonessential nutrients) and others must come from the diet (essential nutrients). A deficiency of either type of nutrient may lead to illness if left untreated.

Antioxidants Give Cell Protection

Antioxidants are essential nutrients that help protect your body against life's stressors. Antioxidant food sources are rich in beta-carotene and vitamins C and E. Antioxidants are thought to play a role in the body's cell-protection system and to interfere with aging and the disease process by neutralizing highly reactive and unstable molecules, called free radicals, produced by the body. In research, free radicals have been shown to disrupt and tear apart vital cell structures like cell membranes. Antioxidants have been shown to tie up these free radicals and take away their destructive power, perhaps reducing the risk of a number of chronic diseases and even slowing the aging process. Eating for wellness requires a diet rich in antioxidants.

Some researchers think that antioxidants might help prevent damage in some types of arthritis and boost immune function when a system is under stress. Both are important benefits for patients.

UNDERSTANDING ANTIOXIDANT FOOD SOURCES

BETA-CAROTENE. Beta-carotene, found in apricots, carrots, cantaloupe, pumpkin, and spinach, is converted to vitamin A in the body. Because of a great deal of media attention, most people think of only beta-carotene as having antioxidant properties, but there are many other carotenoid compounds that do also, including:

alpha-carotene (found in carrots, cantaloupe, and pumpkin)
gamma-carotene (found in apricots and tomatoes)
beta-cryptoxanthin (found in mangoes, nectarines, peaches, and tangerines)
lycopene (found in guava, pink grapefruit, tomatoes, and watermelon)
lutein and zeaxanthin (found in beets, corn, and collard and mustard greens)

SOURCES OF BETA-CAROTENE

apricots	kale
broccoli	papayas
cantaloupes	peaches
carrots	pumpkins
collard greens	red peppers

spinach   turnip greens
sweet potatoes   winter squash
tomatoes

VITAMIN C. Vitamin C (ascorbic acid) protects us against infection and aids in wound healing. When the body is under great stress, the blood levels of ascorbic acid have been found to decline. This decline also occurs with age in both men and women.

Vitamin C plays a vital role in boosting levels of the energizing brain chemical *norepinephrine.* Norepinephrine produces a feeling of alertness and increases concentration. A deficiency of vitamin C can therefore influence your mood as well, leaving you less attentive. It is essential to include plenty of vitamin C sources in your diet.

SOURCES OF VITAMIN C
broccoli   oranges
cantaloupes   peppers
grapefruit and   potatoes
    their juices   strawberries
kiwi   tomatoes

VITAMIN E. Vitamin E is important to the body for the maintenance of cell membranes, and this vitamin's antioxidant effect may slow age-related changes in the body. There is now evidence that vitamin E plays a role in lowering the risk of coronary heart disease and heart attack. Adults with intestinal disorders of malabsorption may be deficient in vitamin E.

Because this vitamin is taken in through vegetables and seed oils, it is difficult to ingest large amounts, especially if you are following a low-fat diet.

If your diet is low in vitamin E food sources, check with your doctor and see if you should add 200 to 400 IU daily.

Supplements can be found at grocery or health food stores
and pharmacies.

SOURCES OF VITAMIN E

margarine   vegetable oils
nuts and seeds   wheat germ

Choose Plant-Based Phytochemicals

Nutrition research is now revealing that a variety of food
choices can do more than provide optimal nutrient intake. A
varied diet can also provide hundreds of nutrient and nonnu-
trient compounds that may be vital to disease protection.
These compounds found in plant-based foods as a group are
referred to as *phytochemicals*.

Phytochemicals appear in all plants. A diet that includes a
variety of grains, fruits, and vegetables should provide these
substances if you vary your choices and methods of food preparation. Although there are phytochemical supplements and
pills, it is better to get your phytochemicals from a varied diet.
Because of the wide array of nutrients in foods essential for

---

TIPS TO BOOST YOUR IMMUNE POWER
- Use a tomato sauce over pasta
- Add tomato sauce to soups and stews
- Add sliced tomatoes to sandwiches and salads
- Add extra vegetables with antioxidants to your dishes
- Throw some greens and carrots in your vegetable soup
- Try a veggie pizza with broccoli and pepper
- Toss some grated zucchini into your next batch of
     muffins or loaf of bread
- Snack on dried fruits and nuts like apricots and cashews
- Use chopped nuts or wheat germ to top off your yogurt

wellness, including those not yet identified, relying on supplements for good nutrition may limit your intake to just known compounds.

A diet for wellness should contain foods loaded with phytochemicals.

PHYTOCHEMICAL FOOD SOURCES

PHYTOCHEMICAL	FOOD SOURCES	WELLNESS FACTOR
Carotenoids	Carrots, apricots, sweet potatoes	Prevent cancer and heart disease
Flavonoids	Apples, onions	Prevent cancer
Indoles	Cruciferous vegetables like cabbage, broccoli, and cauliflower	Prevent breast and uterine cancer
Isoflavones	Legumes, soybeans	Prevent breast and uterine cancer
Lycopene	Tomatoes, red peppers, carrots	Prevent cancer
Sulfides (allyls)	Cabbage, onions, broccoli, garlic, brussels sprouts	Prevent cancer

Five a Day

As you learn to eat for wellness, it is important to follow the nutritional recommendations from the USDA (United States Department of Agriculture), which advises eating five servings of fruits and vegetables a day. Through groundbreaking research, this organization has concluded that we are what we eat, and the nutritional components of fruits and vegetables can prevent or even reverse some diseases and conditions. The National Cancer Institute goes one step beyond the

ADDING PHYTOCHEMICALS TO YOUR DIET
- Use spinach, shredded cabbage, sliced carrots, and broccoli in your salads
- Add chopped fruits to cereal, yogurt, ice cream, and muffins
- Snack on cut-up carrots, pepper, broccoli, and cauliflower
- Make a quick dip by adding tomato salsa to nonfat yogurt
- Fill your pantry with plenty of herbs and spices like ginger, garlic, chives, and parsley
- Frequently include steamed cabbage, broccoli, or brussels sprouts with meals

USDA's recommendation by encouraging us to eat nine servings of fruits and vegetables (or more) a day for better health.

Whether you opt for five a day or can reach the ultimate goal of nine servings a day, it is important to know why this recommendation is important to maintaining good health. The answer lies in the ability of these food sources to prevent a wide range of chronic diseases and bolster the body's immune power. They provide the basic elements for a healthy diet as high-fiber, low-fat powerhouses of antioxidants and phytochemicals, among many other essential and nonessential nutrients.

EASY WAYS TO ADD FRUITS AND VEGETABLES TO YOUR DAILY DIET

Breakfast: 4 oz. of grapefruit juice (1)
1 bagel with jelly
½ cup skim milk

Snack: 1 cup low-fat yogurt
½ cup raspberries (1)

Lunch: ½ cup spinach salad (1)
tuna sandwich with a sliced
tomato (1)
1 cup skim milk

Dinner: ½ cup broccoli (1)
4 oz. baked chicken breast
½ cup wild rice
rolls
½ cup sherbet

TOTAL FOR DAY: 5 servings of fruits and vegetables
To meet the goal for 9 fruits and vegetables a day, increase the amount of salad, vegetables, fruits, and juice to reach the total.

Add Dietary Fiber to Daily Meal Plan

Dietary fiber is one more valuable bonus we get from eating five to nine (or more) servings of fruits or vegetables per day. It is the part of the plant that we can eat but our bodies cannot digest or break down. Fiber moves foods and the toxins they contain quickly through the digestive tract, allowing less time for any possible cancer-causing agents to come in contact with the intestines, colon, or rectum. According to the National Cancer Institute, a diet high in fiber cuts the risk of colon cancer by up to 70 percent and may also lower the risk of kidney and gallstones, as well as ease constipation. Fiber ferments in the colon, increasing the amount of oxygen, which in turn diminishes the action of the harmful bacteria. Fresh, whole fruits and vegetables, including the skins provide the most benefit from fiber. Figs, prunes, pears, and dried beans and peas are also very high in fiber so include them in the diet on a regular basis.

The National Cancer Institute recommends 25 to 35 grams

of fiber per day, yet most Americans eat considerably less than that. About one-fourth of your daily fiber intake should consist of the soluble type fiber found in oats, beans, fruits, and vegetables. The rest of your fiber intake should come from the insoluble type, found in wheat bran and whole grains.

FOODS HIGH IN SOLUBLE FIBER

acorn squash	dates
apples	dried beans
baked potatoes	lentils
blueberries	peas
broccoli	prunes
cabbage	pumpkin
carrots	raspberries
cauliflower	strawberries
citrus fruits	sweet potatoes

You can increase your dietary fiber by adding at least six servings of whole grain breads and cereals, pasta, rice, dried peas, and beans, along with the five to nine servings of fruits and vegetables, to your diet. As you begin to include low-fat, high-complex carbohydrate foods in your diet, you will notice a gradual reduction in your weight. For most patients, this is an appreciated added benefit.

GUIDELINES TO INCREASE FIBER

Eat more legumes that are very high in fiber. Red beans, black beans, great northern beans, and other legumes are high in fiber and have no fat. Don't cook legumes with animal fat.

Eat raw vegetables for snacks. Two carrots will give you a day's supply of vitamin A and provide more than seven grams of fiber.

Read your cereal box at the grocery. If the cereal has less than three grams of fiber, it probably has little nutrient value.

Add dried fruits to your cereal. Three prunes can give you four grams of fiber.

Keep your vegetables crisp when you cook them. Eat them with skins on to add to the fiber content.

Eat fruits with the skin on for an extra fiber boost.

THE FIBER CONTENT OF SELECTED FOODS (GRAMS)	
1 medium bran muffin	3
1 slice of whole wheat toast	2
1 ounce of raisin bran	4
2/3 cup of oatmeal	4.5
1 medium apple with skin	3
1 medium orange	3
1 medium raw carrot	4
1/2 cup of cooked kidney beans	7

Foods for a Calming Effect

As we have discussed above, good nutrition influences our ability to stay healthy and recent research has revealed that what we eat can also affect our moods as well. In the past twenty years, hundreds of studies have confirmed a connection between certain foods and our ability to feel calm and alert. Dr. Judith Wurtman, a nutrition researcher at the Massachusetts Institute of Technology, has found that certain foods affect brain chemicals that influence our mood, mental energy, and performance.

These "persuasive" foods are high in carbohydrates, such as breads, cereal, pasta, or sherbet, and raise the level of serotonin in the brain. When serotonin levels rise, we feel calm and upbeat for a period of time. As discussed throughout the book, serotonin is the mood-elevating neurotransmitter; it plays an unknown role in fibromyalgia symptoms, especially with depression and sleep disorders. Studies have shown that by including plenty of foods high in complex carbohydrates in your diet, you can boost the level of serotonin and reap the benefits of feeling calm throughout the day and sleeping more soundly at night.

Even though we have a host of new information on the food-mood connection, finding foods that relieve depressed feelings relies on a personal trial-and-error approach. Using the list of the suggested serotonin-boosting foods below, see which ones make a difference in your symptoms and wellness, then incorporate these in five to six minimeals throughout the day to keep blood sugar and energy levels even.

HIGH-CARBOHYDRATE FOODS THAT BOOST SEROTONIN

bagels	pasta
bread	potatoes
cereal	rice
crackers	sherbet
muffins	

Foods to Boost Energy and Alertness

Just as some foods can be used to create a calm feeling during times when you experience great stress or anxiety, other foods can create the opposite effect, making you feel attentive and responsive. Foods rich in protein, like turkey, tuna, or chicken, are also rich in an amino acid called tyrosine. Tyrosine boosts levels of the neurotransmitters dopamine and norepinephrine. Neurotransmitters are the chemicals that get messages from cell to cell. Sophisticated research by Dr. Judith Wurtman at MIT has revealed that people are more alert when the brain is producing the neurotransmitters dopamine and norepinephrine. The neurotransmitter serotonin is associated with less anxiety and increased drowsiness. Dopamine and norepinephrine may be produced through the dietary consumption of protein. When we eat protein food, this increases the amino acid tyrosine, which boosts the levels of dopamine and norepinephrine. This, in turn, creates a feeling of alertness and improves our concentration. A protein source should be included in your diet several times a day, especially during those times when you need to clear your mind and boost your energy.

Try the following to see which foods boost stamina and alertness.

HIGH-PROTEIN FOODS RICH IN TYROSINE

beans and peas	soy products (soy
beef	beans, soy
cheese	granules, soy
fish	milk, etc.)
milk	yogurt
poultry	

Repairing the Damage of Fibromyalgia

Protein is also important in building and repairing body tissue and in fighting infection. Too little protein in the diet may lead to symptoms of fatigue, weakness, apathy, and poor immunity. The average-size adult needs 45 to 55 grams of protein a day. More protein is needed if there is fever or infection.

One ounce of meat, chicken, cheese, or fish provides 7 grams of protein; 1 cup of milk provides 8 grams of protein. Therefore 5 to 6 ounces of meat per day and 2 cups of milk provide adequate protein for most adults. Vegetable proteins can make a good substitute for animal protein, if eaten with a complementary starch at the same meal. An example of this would be to substitute 1½ cups of black beans and rice for a 2-ounce portion of meat.

COMPLEMENTARY VEGETABLE PROTEINS

beans and bread
beans and rice
corn tortillas and
   beans

legumes and
   grains
peanut butter
   and bread

Include Iron-Rich Foods

Some specific nutrient deficiencies can impact on how you feel. For example, if you are not including iron-rich foods in your diet (especially menstruating women), then iron-deficiency anemia can result. Symptoms of fatigue, weakness, shortness of breath, and pallor can compound symptoms of fibromyalgia. Make sure your diet includes plenty of iron-rich foods.

IRON-RICH FOODS

dried apricots
dried beans
enriched or fortified bread and cereals
lean, fat-trimmed cuts of red meat (beef, veal, or lamb)
lentils
prunes
raisins

When eating an iron-rich food from a plant source, include a vitamin C source, such as orange or grapefruit juice, along with it to enhance iron absorption. Vitamin C–fortified apple juice is also a good source.

Minimize PMS with Nutritional and Activity Changes

Because female patients with fibromyalgia tend to suffer with painful menstrual cramps, it is important to minimize premenstrual syndrome (PMS) symptoms through some dietary and activity changes. PMS symptoms may include mild breast tenderness, fluid retention, anxiety, dietary cravings, irritability, and an inability to concentrate. Unfortunately, neither the cause nor the cure for PMS is currently known. However, these measures may help alleviate some of the symptoms.

Eat a balanced diet that includes a variety of complex carbohydrate foods (grains, fruits, and vegetables) and a moderate amount of meat and milk products.

Exercise regularly to reduce stress and keep your body fit. A daily exercise program can decrease PMS symptoms. This lessening of symptoms may be connected with the rise in endorphins that occurs with an intense aerobic workout. Regular aerobic exercise increases one's sense of well-being and decreases fluid retention. It has also been shown to be effective in the treatment of depression.

Avoid alcohol before your menstrual period. Since alcohol is a mood-altering drug, it can compound feelings of depression and hopelessness. Furthermore, many women have a decreased tolerance for alcohol prior to their period and they may become intoxicated quickly.

Avoid caffeine before and during your menstrual period. Studies have shown that symptoms of PMS in-

creased with the consumption of caffeine-containing beverages. In one study, women who totally abstained from caffeine had a complete resolution of symptoms from PMS.

Reduce excessive sodium and salt in the diet to reduce fluid retention. Excessive sodium can lead to bloating, edema, and fluid weight gain during premenstruation; reducing the sodium in the diet can relieve some of these symptoms. The best approach is to eat more foods naturally low in sodium. This includes fresh fruits and vegetables, cereals, and grains. Another way is to limit the consumption of high-sodium processed foods and the use of table salt. You can add a splash of lemon juice to a glass of water for a natural diuretic.

If you experience premenstrual symptoms of *hypoglycemia* (low blood sugar), such as fatigue, dizziness, and the shakes, divide your meals into six small minimeals rich in complex carbohydrates and protein and low in simple sugars. (For lists of foods high in complex carbohydrates and protein see pages 136 to 138.)

FOODS HIGH IN SIMPLE SUGARS
cakes
candy and gum
canned fruits in syrup
cookies
frozen yogurt and sherbet
fruit juice
pies
regular sodas and sweetened drinks

FOODS HIGH IN SODIUM
canned meats
canned soups
canned tomato products
canned vegetables
frozen prepared meals (vegetables with sauces, meats, cas-
    seroles)
processed meats
salted snacks, such as chips, peanuts, pretzels

Vitamin Supplements

Various vitamins and minerals have also been suggested as
effective for treatment of chronic muscle pain. No specific
evidence favors any single vitamin or mineral supplement, but
if you are in doubt, talk with your physician or licensed nutritionist. Premenopausal women especially need to check for
iron deficiency. Even a mild deficiency in iron can make it
difficult to get through the day without overwhelming fatigue.

If you do take vitamins to boost your immune power, start
with a multiple vitamin without minerals that has the Recommended Daily Allowance (RDA) as suggested by the American Dietetics Association, then talk with a nutritionist about
your specific vitamin needs.

Omega-3

Some foods have been shown to decrease inflammation in
the body, while others tend to increase the possibility of inflammation. For example, animal foods contain fats that
have been found to increase an inflammatory response. But
studies show that eating high-fat fish, such as mackerel,
bluefish, or tuna, that contain N-3 or omega-3 fatty acids
enables the body to make products that tend to decrease
the inflammation.

The most commonly available of these omega-3 fatty acids is found in some fish and fish oil. Although guidelines have not been established regarding supplements of fish oil, EPA (eicosapentaenoic acid) is available in capsules without a prescription. You can ask for these capsules at your drugstore or health food store. Check the instructions on the label as to suggested dosage.

Some patients with arthritis have found improvement in pain and stiffness when they take these capsules for a few months. It is important to use EPA in addition to your basic treatment program, not in replacement of it. When used in the dosage prescribed on the label, no serious side effects are known.

Vegetarians who want to gain this anti-inflammatory benefit can substitute borage seed oil, flaxseed oil, blackcurrant seed oil (BCSO), or evening primrose oil—all said to be helpful in offsetting the inflammation caused by arthritis. These oils all contain gammalinolenic acid (GLA), an omega-6 oil. One study of patients with active rheumatoid arthritis found that BCSO is a potentially effective treatment. Similar studies with fibromyalgia patients have not yet been conclusive.

FISH HIGH IN OMEGA-3

anchovies	salmon
bluefish	sardines
capeline	shad
dogfish	sturgeon
herring	tuna
mackerel	whitefish

An Alkaline Diet

The arthritis diet is an alkaline diet used by some patients for the treatment of osteoarthritis, rheumatoid arthritis, and other conditions where overacidity is thought to play a part. Naturo-paths believe that arthritis is caused by the accumulation of toxic acids in the joints. These acids are thought to come naturally from the intestine, and from a failure of the body's metabolism to detoxify them when in excess in the diet. While dietary changes, such as following a vegetarian diet, have proven to be helpful for patients with rheumatoid arthritis, studies are still inconclusive for those with fibromyalgia.

A Fibromyalgia Diet?

Some people with fibromyalgia find that highly acidic foods, such as citrus products, foods in the nightshade family (to-mato products, potatoes, eggplant, peppers, tobacco), red meat, cow's milk products, brown and white wheat flour products, sugar-containing foods, coffee, chocolate, and honey, seem to trigger more muscle pain. Eliminating foods to reduce pain is strictly personal and must be done on a case-by-case basis.

If you do try a food-restrictive diet, such as the one offered here, be sure to check with your physician or nutritionist about nutrient supplements that you may need.

AN ALKALINE DIET FOR ARTHRITIS

Foods to Avoid	Foods to Eat
Red meat	White fish, lentils, peas, chicken, eggs (no more than 4 per week)
Cow's milk, cheese, and yogurt	Goat's milk, cheese, soy milk
Brown, white, wheat flour	Oats, brown rice, corn, buckwheat,

Citrus fruit

millet, 100% rye
crispbread
Tomatoes (no more than
twice a week),
all other fruit, all
vegetables

FOODS TO AVOID
Dry roasted nuts

Sugar and foods
containing sugar,
syrup, honey
Coffee, decaf coffee,
cocoa, tea, alcohol

Salt, pepper, vinegar

Butter and margarine
Chocolate

FOODS TO EAT
All other nuts, especially
hazelnut, almond,
cashew, and walnut
Sugarcane, molasses,
dried fruit, sugar-free
products
Grain coffees, herbal
teas, unsweetened
fruit juices, vegetable
juices
Ruthmol salt, cubes of
vegetarian stock
Vegetable oil
Carob

In short, good nutrition can help you take an active role in
your health and healing. While there are no guarantees that
the foods you eat will heal your fibromyalgia, we do know that
good nutrition offers tremendous benefits of increased energy
and boosts your immune system to the point where it can
cope with the symptoms and fight off other serious illnesses.

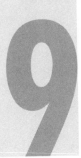

STEP 7:
SEEK SUPPORT

Living with fibromyalgia is not easy. You may often feel that no one understands the pain, fatigue, and stress that you feel twenty-four hours a day, month after month, year after year. If prolonged, these overwhelming feelings of isolation can become a stumbling block in your quest for wellness, resulting in increased stress, anxiety, and difficulty obtaining restful sleep, not to mention difficulty in keeping healthy relationships.

It does not have to be this way. You can and must seek support to keep fibromyalgia symptoms under control and to feel whole. Whether your main support comes from your physician, a personal friend, a support group of fibromyalgia patients, or even strangers on the Internet, there are caring contacts available—if you seek them.

See an Arthritis Specialist, If Needed

Because fibromyalgia is a rheumatic disease like arthritis, obtaining proper help begins with a specific and accurate diagnosis from a physician who understands the syndrome. I suggest that you start with your primary physician, then, if needed, seek confirmation from a board-certified rheumatologist, a specialist who diagnoses and treats fibromyalgia daily.

Beyond the initial diagnosis are a host of professionals, from physical therapists and psychologists to sleep disorder specialists and dietitians, who can help you implement the 7-Step Treatment Program as defined in this book.

Consider a Fibromyalgia Support Group

Everyone needs someone to talk to. It may be a good idea to branch out and join a fibromyalgia support group as you experience give-and-take with other sufferers.

Support is necessary for coping with any chronic illness. A support group is geared toward the unique needs of its members and is especially important for fibromyalgia patients. While support groups are not psychotherapy groups, they do provide patients with a safe and accepting place to vent their frustrations, share their situations, and receive comfort and encouragement from one another. In many such groups, the latest methods of treatment are discussed and members give coping suggestions that you may not be aware of. Assurance is given that someone else knows what you are going through, as people share their struggles in living with this mysterious syndrome. This camaraderie is necessary in order to help you revamp your thought processes. After joining such a group, you may realize that the best experts on a disease are often those who live with it daily, although you should always check with your physician before taking a new remedy.

Fibromyalgia support groups are active around the world. Call the Fibromyalgia Association or the Arthritis Foundation (numbers listed on page 153) for more information on support groups in your area. You may also check with your physician or local hospitals to see if such groups are registered. If you cannot find a group, the Fibromyalgia Association or Arthritis

Foundation can provide you with information on how to start one yourself.

Try Internet Support Groups

If you would prefer not to join a group, you can find support in the privacy of your home or office on the Internet. You can exchange E-mail with those in foreign countries, who may, in turn, suggest excellent remedies that may not be popular in the United States. When going on-line, check into the World Wide Web for the latest information on fibromyalgia, along with current periodicals and studies on the disease.

On the World Wide Web, you can visit the USA Fibrositis Association home page and the Fibromyalgia news group, among many.

Seek Support from Loved Ones

"I know she is sick, but to be honest, she looks very healthy to me." Tom came to see me about his wife, Claire, to try to find more information on fibromyalgia.

"My boss thinks I'm lazy," Ellen cried during a recent appointment after living with this disease for three years. "I cannot convince him that even though I look normal on the outside, I'm far from being normal on the inside."

Fibromyalgia's reach extends beyond the patient and can affect the entire family. Especially with such a chronic pain–related disease, personal support is necessary, whether from your spouse, family, friends, or coworkers.

It is important to educate your friends and loved ones about your disease, sensitizing them to the symptoms that may come and go but which can be immobilizing at times. I have found that not only should the patient be told how to treat this disease, but it is helpful to explain the protocol for treatment to those close to the patient.

Family members can have the best of intentions, but without specific guidance, they sometimes make things worse. Family meetings with a licensed mental health counselor are another way of helping everyone deal with the stress of your disease and may be necessary if lifestyle changes have to be made to accommodate your problems.

Consider a Comprehensive Pain Clinic

If you are still having great pain after months of using the suggested 7-Step Treatment Program in this book, it may be necessary to seek additional support from a comprehensive pain clinic.

Most pain clinics use a multidisciplinary approach to treatment, including medical treatment, physical therapy, and psychological approaches to pain control. As you have learned by reading this book, each of these areas is important and complements the others.

Health care specialists at comprehensive pain clinics usually see more severe cases of deep muscle pain since, by the time of admission, most patients have tried a myriad of other treatments. Even with these more difficult cases, many comprehensive pain clinics across the nation are finding that patients are twice as likely to return to work after comprehensive pain treatment than after other treatments alone. In fact, 40 to 60 percent of the patients with chronic pain treated in comprehensive clinics return to work and report having less pain and improved activity. Considering that these patients had not responded to most other treatment, the figures are encouraging.

HOW TO CHOOSE A PAIN UNIT

The American Chronic Pain Association recommends considering the following guidelines prior to selecting a pain unit. You can contact this organization at P.O. Box 850, Rocklin, CA 95677 or call (916) 632-0922. Your personal physician can refer you to a unit, but many programs accept self-referral.

1. Make sure you locate a legitimate program. Facilities that offer pain management should include several specific components, listed below.
- The Commission on Accreditation of Rehabilitation Facilities (CARF) (telephone: [800] 444-8991) can provide you with a listing of accredited pain programs in your area (your health insurance may require that the unit be CARF-accredited in order for you to receive reimbursement).
- You can also contact the American Pain Society, a group of health care providers, at (708) 966-5595 for additional information about pain units in your area.

2. Choose a good program that is convenient for you and your family.
- Many pain-management programs do not offer outpatient care. Choosing a program close to your home will enable you to commute to the program each day.

3. Learn something about the people who run the program.
- Try to meet several of the staff members to get a sense of the people you will be dealing with while on the unit.
- The program should have a complete medical staff trained in pain-management techniques including:
  - ✓ Physician (may be a specialist from several different areas but should have expertise in pain management)
  - ✓ Registered nurse

√ Psychiatrist or psychologist
√ Physical therapist
√ Occupational therapist
√ Biofeedback therapist
√ Family counselor
√ Vocational counselor
√ Personnel trained in pain-management intervention

4. Make sure the program includes most of the following features:

Biofeedback training
Counseling
Family counseling
TENS (Transcutaneous Electrical Nerve Stimulation) units
Group therapy
Occupational therapy
Assertiveness training
Regional anesthesia (nerve blocks)
Physical therapy (exercise and body mechanics training, not massage, whirlpool, etc.)
Relaxation training and stress management
Educational program covering medications and other aspects of pain and its management
Aftercare (follow-up support once you have left the unit)

5. Be sure your family can be involved in your care.
• Family members should be required to be involved in your treatment.
• If you choose an out-of-town unit, find out if your family can be involved in your care.
• The program should provide special educational sessions for family members.
• Joint counseling for you and your family should also be available.

6. Also consider these additional factors:

- What services will your insurance company reimburse, and what will you be expected to cover?
- What is the unit's physical setup (is it in a patient care area or in an area by itself)?
- Is the program inpatient or outpatient (when going through medication detoxification, inpatient care is recommended)?
- Do you understand what will be required of you during your stay (length of time you will be on unit, responsibility to take care of personal needs, etc.)?
- Does the unit provide any type of job retraining?
- Make sure that, before accepting you, the unit reviews your previous medical records and gives you a complete physical evaluation to be sure you can participate in the program.
- Obtain copies of your recent medical records to prevent duplicate testing.
- Try to talk with both present and past program participants to get their feedback about their stay on the unit.

Consider the expense before you go to a pain clinic. It should be the last resort with fibromyalgia and considered only if all other methods of treatment fail.

Seeking Support with a Therapist

The fibromyalgia patient deals with pain on a daily basis and the reason for the pain is genuine—there is something wrong in the body. For most people, the last thing you want to hear is, "I think it might be a good idea for you to speak with someone about the depression and stress you have." You may conclude that the "someone" is either a psychiatrist, psychologist, or a counselor of some type—a "shrink." You may be offended by the implication that the disease is "in your head." You may even become suspicious that this person does not believe that you are really feeling the pain and fatigue that you describe.

It is a fact that all people with pain, whether from fibromyalgia or other diseases, have stress, which in turn makes it more difficult to handle everyday issues, much less crisis situations that may arise. One fibromyalgia patient, Sandra, who had severe muscle pain in her shoulders, described her personality as "Dr. Jekyll and Mr. Hyde."

"Depending on whether I've slept well or not, my personality changes with the wind. I warn family and friends not to take offense when I come across irritable or irrational," she said.

Psychological counseling can help you develop appropriate and workable coping strategies to deal with the issues that affect you. It is an accepted treatment for anyone—not just people who have psychological problems or diseases.

If you do seek psychological intervention, not only will you learn new coping methods, but you will also obtain the much-needed support of a professional who understands your feelings and emotions. It is most helpful if your therapist is trained in the area of pain management and / or fibromyalgia.

You may select a one-on-one session with a therapist. These sessions may include specific help with alleviating depression, anxiety, or stress, along with many other problem areas addressed more specifically in the following section. Other sessions may include a meeting with family members or a group session, such as a support group.

Information Organizations and Support Groups

There is also support available from numerous organizations across the nation. These groups can provide you with brochures on fibromyalgia and related problems and assist you with finding a physician, support group, or pain clinic, if needed.

Advil Forum on
  Healthcare
1500 Broadway, 26th Floor
New York, NY 10036
*Ask for a brochure on pain
  relief for back pain or
  arthritis.*

Aids for Arthritis
3 Little Knoll Court
Medford, NJ 08055
(609) 654-6918

American Chronic Pain
  Association
P.O. Box 850
Rocklin, CA 95677
(916) 632-0922

Arthritis Foundation
1314 Spring Street
Atlanta, GA 30309
(800) 283-7800
(404) 872-7100

Arthritis Society
250 Floor Street East, Suite
  901
Toronto, Ontario
CANADA M4W 3P2
(416) 967-1414

Fibromyalgia Association
P.O. Box 21988
Columbus, OH 43221-0988
(614) 457-4222 (phone)
(614) 457-2729 (fax)

Fibromyalgia Network
5700 Stockdale Highway,
  Suite 100
Bakersfield, CA 93309
(805) 631-1950

Help for Incontinent People
P.O. Box 544
Union, SC 29379

Managing Medications
Dept. S
P.O. Box 15329
Stamford, CT 06901
*Send a self-addressed
  stamped envelope for
  information on
  recognizing adverse drug
  reactions.*

National Arthritis &
  Musculoskeletal & Skin
  Diseases Information
  Clearinghouse
One AMS Circle
Bethesda, MD 20892-3675
(301) 495-4484

National Chronic Fatigue
    Syndrome and
    Fibromyalgia Association
3521 Broadway, Suite 222
Kansas City, MO 64111
(816) 931-4777

National Headache
    Foundation
(800) 843-2256

National Mental Health
    Association
(800) 969-6642

The pressures of living with a chronic disease can overwhelm you, but it does not have to be this way, as support is available. Ask your doctor to recommend professional help and resources, including psychologists, support groups, or other patients who have fibromyalgia and want to help others. Send away for pamphlets and brochures from national organizations listed in this chapter, or go on-line and plug into a support group on the Internet.

Support from others can help you realize that you are not alone in dealing with fibromyalgia and can give new confidence as you learn to handle the daily challenges in a reasonable manner.

10
QUESTIONS PATIENTS ASK ABOUT FIBROMYALGIA

I believe that learning from others who have fibromyalgia is an excellent way to gain control over the disease's long-lasting symptoms. The following commonly asked questions will reinforce your understanding of the disease and the practical and medical responses for coping that you've learned from this book.

Q. After living with fibromyalgia symptoms for six years, my doctor recently diagnosed it as a specific disease. She sent me to a fibromyalgia support group in our city, and thirty-two of the thirty-eight members were women around my age (age forty-nine). Does this mean that fibromyalgia is a middle-aged woman's disease?

A. It is really common to be bothered by the feelings of fibromyalgia for years before an exact diagnosis is made. Once the diagnosis is made, however, the picture becomes clear. Only then can proper treatment begin.

Support groups for fibromyalgia are a great source of information. This is a good way to keep up with the latest research and treatments available. Dealing with fibromyalgia alone can be discouraging; it helps to talk openly with others who have dealt with the problem successfully. Also, you may be able to help others.

Yes, it is a fact that most fibromyalgia patients are women, but it can happen in men. About 90 percent of patients (nine in ten) are women, commonly in the middle years of life.

Q. I keep hearing that this is a woman's disease, yet I am a 6'2" male who was recently diagnosed with fibromyalgia. Could there be a hormonal problem that is causing this to happen to my body? If so, what treatment would be effective?

A. While it is true that the vast majority of cases of fibromyalgia happen in women, it is also true that men suffer from this disease as well. The specific causes are not known. In our clinic, we do see fibromyalgia in men at times and some of them have had a severe injury to the back, such as a ruptured disc in the lumbar spine, months or even years before.

There is no evidence that hormones play a role in fibromyalgia in men. The treatment is the same for both men and women and by staying on my 7-Step Treatment Program, you should obtain relief.

Q. I was diagnosed with fibromyalgia after having great pain stemming from a hysterectomy. I had pain when I awoke, then more pain throughout the day. Then it seemed as if my bladder completely shut down. I was rushed to the emergency room for a catheterization and was told it was part of fibromyalgia. Have you ever heard of this happening?

A. Fibromyalgia can begin after a very stressful situation, an injury, or a serious illness. Some women have found that it began after a hysterectomy. Remember, the causes are just not known. Many problems other than pain and stiffness can result, such as abdominal pain, bloating, constipation and diarrhea, and irritable bowel syndrome (IBS).

Also, as discussed on page 21, urinary frequency, the urge to urinate, and pain on urination can come with fibromyalgia. There is no special treatment other than the treatment of the disease itself and certain medicines that can help the bladder control.

Talk to your doctor to be sure you have the best combination of medicines to control the symptoms of this disease.

Q. My family practitioner is treating me for fibromyalgia, but I feel that I need a specialist. What type of doctor would you recommend for this disease? Are there certain tests I will need?

A. See your family doctor first, but if your fibromyalgia is not improved after a reasonable amount of time (say a few months), then yes, it is a good idea to ask for an opinion from a rheumatologist. Rheumatologists deal with arthritis and related diseases. They treat many patients with fibromyalgia. This specialist will review your diagnosis and coordinate the plan for treatment.

The diagnosis of fibromyalgia is still made from an examination and talking with the patient. A few blood tests and X rays will help to eliminate other types of arthritis. This is important to be sure that no other specific treatments will be needed. If the rheumatologist agrees with the diagnosis of fibromyalgia, a plan for treatment can be made.

Q. After a lengthy bout with the flu, my seventeen-year-old daughter was diagnosed with fibromyalgia. Is this common?

A. Fibromyalgia does happen in teenagers. While uncommon, it causes the same pain, stiffness, and fatigue that adults experience. It usually improves slowly over time. The course of treatment may be helped by a regular program of moist heat, exercises, and medication as discussed in chapter 3. Just as in adults, fibromyalgia in teenagers seems to follow a severe injury or illness, but the exact reason why is not known.

Q. Does taking estrogen have anything to do with fibromyalgia? After a complete hysterectomy at age thirty-five, my doctor put me on estrogen replacement. Within one year, I developed horrible muscle pain and fatigue that would not end, even with bed rest. Was it the estrogen? If so, what should I do?

A. There is no good evidence that the hysterectomy or the estrogen treatment are the cause of fibromyalgia, although fibromyalgia does occur in some women after a hysterectomy. The surgery as well as the estrogen treatment are common events in many women. Unless your doctor advises otherwise, you can continue your estrogen treatment without fear of aggravating your fibromyalgia.

However, in some patients with fibromyalgia, there does seem to be a major illness, injury, or emotional stress just before the start of their symptoms. It is not known how these events seem to trigger fibromyalgia. Perhaps future research will bring this answer to light.

Q. Fibromyalgia has taken over my life and is taking over my family's life as well. Is there a cure for this or will it continue to cause pain forever? Growing older with all this pain does not seem appealing. What does research show for the future?

A. The chronic pain and fatigue can certainly take over your life. It can cause avoidance of your usual activities, less exercise, more pain, and a vicious cycle of further withdrawal, which can lead to depression. The chronic pain of fibromyalgia can change your personality, making it difficult to get along with those you love.

Although there is no cure and no prediction about how long the disease will take to run its course, it's important that your family shares in your disease. When you are tired, stressed, and in pain, it affects how your family feels and acts.

A big problem in fibromyalgia is that the patient does not appear to be sick. There are few outward signs of pain. The frustration from your inability to keep up with your activities shows to others in the way you act. It is a good idea to see a clinical psychologist or psychiatrist for tips on stress management. This professional can be invaluable in helping you deal with the stress of chronic pain.

Right now, there is no cure for fibromyalgia in sight, but good treatment is available and will work, if you stick to the 7-Step Program. Most patients eventually improve with treatment. Your goals might be to have a reasonable relief of the pain and tiredness so that you can get around and do the things you need to do each day.

Q. I am the mother of three daughters and was recently diagnosed with fibromyalgia. Does this mean that my daughters will also be subject to this disease? Are there prevention methods?

A. If you have the diagnosis of fibromyalgia, it does not mean that your daughters are also destined to be sufferers. The causes of fibromyalgia are unknown. Since there are no known ways to prevent fibromyalgia, I suggest that you simply keep up a good exercise program, including maintaining your cardiovascular fitness, and encourage your daughters to do the same. There is some evidence that an ongoing exercise program, including good conditioning, may make a person more resistant to fibromyalgia.

Q. I started the daily exercise program, but on some days just getting out of bed is a chore. Then, after I exercise, I ache even more. Should I push myself even when the pain and fatigue are unbearable?

A. Most patients with fibromyalgia feel stiff on awakening in the morning. It may even take an hour or more to loosen up. These feelings are very much a part of the disease. Usually, when there is relief of other symptoms with treatment, there is also improvement in the morning stiffness.

It is also typical to have worsening of the aching and pain after exercise. This is a big problem, since it can make patients avoid exercise, an important healing component of the 7-Step Treatment Program. In our clinic, we suggest that patients do their best to keep up the regular exercise program, on good and bad days.

Aerobic exercise, such as an exercise class, walking, bicycling, or swimming, should be continued daily, if possible. On bad days, you might do a little less, but try not to stop completely. Gradually increase back to your old level as soon as you feel less pain.

Remember, on days when you feel better, you may be tempted to totally skip exercise. Don't let this happen! Regular exercise can help you have more good days in the future.

Q. I started NSAIDs for the muscle aches of fibromyalgia, but they did little for the pain. Without purchasing a host of medications, is there a way to tell which medication will help most?

A. NSAIDs (nonsteroidal anti-inflammatory medications) may not help at all in fibromyalgia. This is because there is little inflammation present in the tissues, if fibromyalgia is the only problem. But these medications may also be used as pain relievers, so you may try them for that reason.

There are more than twenty NSAIDs available on the market. Most people find one that works without side effects, but it may be necessary to try a number of different types to find the one that is best. Ask your doctor to make a suggestion. In our clinic we try to provide our patients with manufacturer samples. When a patient finds a sample medication that works effectively, then the medication can be purchased.

If you notice any new problems, such as nausea, then check with your doctor to see if you should continue using this NSAID.

Q. My doctor told me that my constant pain and fatigue were caused by fibromyalgia, even though my lab tests were normal. How can she be sure that this is fibromyalgia and not some other disease?

A. There are no specific blood tests or other tests that can definitely make the diagnosis of fibromyalgia, but these tests can help rule out certain diseases. The diagnosis is made by the symptoms you express to your doctor: the widespread pain, the trigger points, typical fatigue, depression, and other problems as discussed in chapter 2. Some of the most common problems that may also be present with fibromyalgia include osteoarthritis, rheumatoid arthritis, and other types of arthritis or thyroid disease. Each of these problems has specific symptoms and tests for diagnosis.

Q. Can't I speed up the course of fibromyalgia? I've had this disease for seven years and see no end in sight.

A. Fibromyalgia can last for years, but there are definite steps you can take to control the symptoms. There is no cure at this time, but the program of moist heat, exercises, medication, and other measures can make the pain tolerable. If you can control your pain and do most of your usual activities, you can win against fibromyalgia.

Many researchers have found that after a few years, the limitations from fibromyalgia are fewer. Many people still have some pain but not the severe and widespread pain and fatigue that was present in earlier years. One study found 24 percent of patients developed excellent control of their symptoms. About 50 percent of patients in the same study experienced more frequent pain-free periods. You can speed up the improvement of the disease with the 7-Step Treatment Program as described in this book.

Q. What about moist heat in the treatment of fibromyalgia? I bought a Jacuzzi in hopes that this would help alleviate my constant pain.

A. I don't know of anyone who has not felt totally relaxed after spending time in a Jacuzzi or whirlpool bath. Hot baths are part of one of the oldest methods of alternative treatments for chronic pain associated with arthritis, specifically fibromyalgia. The Romans built baths to provide warm pools for treatment, and the theory behind these baths is just as useful today. The moist heat gives soothing relief to painful muscle aches and provides comfort just as in today's treatments. Many times after relaxing in a whirlpool or Jacuzzi, you are able to do your exercises easily, without as much muscle pain.

Q. Why do you keep saying to exercise when I can hardly get out of the chair? I cannot imagine starting a walking or biking program with the pain I have.

A. Many researchers find exercise to be one of the most important parts of the treatment of fibromyalgia, because it can help improve endurance and strength. Most fibromyalgia patients have not exercised regularly for some time because of the pain and are out of condition. However, in treating hundreds of patients with fibromyalgia, we have learned that those who start and continue an exercise program are much more likely to see their symptoms improve.

Usually, the most difficult part is starting the exercise

program when you are stiff and in pain. Two types of exercise are helpful. One is endurance exercise, which gives good cardiovascular exercise and improves fitness. This can improve your ability to accomplish daily activities, reduce stress and anxiety, and help with depression.

How do you start endurance exercise? Simply make yourself start walking every day. Walk a short distance, one that you can easily accomplish, and gradually increase that distance. Or use an electronic treadmill indoors and slowly increase the time you spend on the machine.

The second type of exercise used to treat fibromyalgia is muscle-strengthening exercise. These simple exercises, described in chapter 4, can be done at home. Muscle-strengthening exercise achieves two goals: Stronger and more flexible muscles are less likely to become painful and stiff with daily activity; and stronger muscles are less likely to become tired and fatigued with activity.

Q. A friend of mine who also has fibromyalgia mentioned trying DMSO for pain relief. What is DMSO and how is it used? Is it safe?

A. DMSO (dimethyl sulfoxide) is sold in an impure form in some hardware stores and has been used to treat illnesses in horses for years. In humans, DMSO has been used by athletes to treat injuries to muscles and tendons. It is a liquid that is absorbed into the system when applied to the skin. Side effects include strong, garlicky breath odor and occasional skin irritation where it was applied. If DMSO is injected into a vein, it is very dangerous and can cause liver and other internal organ damage. This should never be done.

While the U.S. Food and Drug Administration (FDA) has not approved DMSO for use in treating arthritis or bursitis, it has found that it might be helpful in relieving pain caused by bursitis, acute injuries, and possibly rheu-

matoid arthritis. DMSO is used by some fibromyalgia patients. In my clinic, I see little use among fibromyalgia
patients, but I do not object if it is used carefully and gives
relief.

Q. What about usage of over-the-counter creams, liniments,
and lotions for muscle pain relief with fibromyalgia? Are
these harmful?

A. Creams, liniments, and lotions are widely advertised and
used for the pain of arthritis and other conditions. Many
types are available at your drugstore and at health food
stores. They are not harmful when used properly and can
be continued if you feel improvement in muscle pain.

One newer topical cream, capsaicin, sold over the
counter under various brand names, such as Capsaicin or
Zostrix, has been found to be quite beneficial in the few
existing studies. One particular capsaicin lotion is available
in a roll-on applicator and is sold as Capsin (ask your pharmacist for information on this product).

Capsaicin has an active ingredient derived from red chili
peppers. When nerve endings in the body are touched by
capsaicin, they produce *substance P,* a neurotransmitter
that carries pain messages to the brain. Repeated applica-
tions of capsaicin results in fewer pain messages to the
brain. While this cream can cause warmth or a burning
sensation, it does not cause blistering, and the burning
feeling usually decreases the longer the cream is used.

Q. My friend told me about a cream that is only found at
health food stores that is made from an herb. Do you
know anything about this?

A. Boswellian Cream can be found at some health food stores
and has been used for centuries to treat pain-related ailments. This cream is made of four triterpene acids from
the herb *Boswellia serrata,* which has been found to bring

temporary relief to minor aches and pains associated with arthritis.

Use this cream with caution, as it does produce mild inflammation and redness to the skin when applied, supposedly in order to achieve its healing properties. A loose bandage should be applied after the cream. Boswellian Cream is for external use only; if your skin becomes inflamed, stop its usage.

Q. I'm trying to use complementary treatments in controlling stress. More specifically, I've started a regular program of guided imagery, along with progressive relaxation and deep breathing. How will I know if this is working?

A. Each person reacts differently, and some forms of mind / body therapy will be successful in some patients and less useful in others. The best results happen when the most effective methods for each patient are used for symptom relief. As always, everyone is different. The important factor is to choose those that work for you and launch out in a regular, daily program of relaxation. Monitor your heart rate as you do this. Does the relaxation help you feel calm and at ease? Continue to practice the technique(s) that you choose until you are able to elicit the relaxation response anytime during the day, especially during stressful moments.

Q. You keep emphasizing the importance of a "combination" treatment program. What exactly does this mean?

A. Let me answer that by using two interesting case studies. Patty epitomized the typical fibromyalgia patient. This thirty-seven-year-old mother maintained a very successful home-based business while caring for her four children. She volunteered at her church and helped teach computer at her children's school two afternoons a week. While she never found time to exercise, Patty was able to maintain a normal weight simply from the nervous energy she burned balancing so many responsibilities . . . until she was diagnosed with fibromyalgia.

"It started with unending fatigue after getting the flu last winter," she said. "I kept thinking that if only I could get more sleep I would feel well, but the tiredness wouldn't go away. Then I began to feel achy all over, day after day. Sometimes I got a grinding sound in my neck when I moved it. My neck began to feel stiff all the time, as well as both shoulders, and when I touched my neck, it felt warm. My muscles would be so sore that it felt like I had exercised for hours the day before, but I hadn't. Even my scalp hurt."

Patty didn't have time to tolerate the interruption of fibromyalgia's symptoms in her busy life. I recommended her to a stress clinic in town, where she worked with the therapists using biofeedback, guided imagery, and the relaxation response. Her physical therapist referred her to a licensed massage therapist, and she went for weekly muscle massages. After three months of treatment, medication that helped her to achieve restful sleep, and a regular exercise program, Patty was feeling hopeful that she could live a normal life in spite of her disease.

Patty's experience illustrates what I have found to be true, that a combination treatment program can assist a patient in decreasing stress and pacing her lifestyle so that the symptoms of fibromyalgia are diminished or managed.

When forty-six-year-old Marilyn came to see me for an evaluation, she had experienced fibromyalgia symptoms for three years. "The symptoms began around the time my last son left for college," she told me. "At that time, I was very anxious and mildly depressed. My husband, Ray, was fully involved in his career and both boys were away at school. All I had to occupy my time was cleaning the house each day and waiting for Ray to come home from work."

Marilyn told of feeling stiffness and pain in her arms and hands, especially her right hand and thumb. She also had a pinching pain in her left hip, making it difficult to lift her foot to walk. Fibromyalgia also caused painful cramps and sharp, stabbing pains in her left calf. Her toes on the same side would suddenly pull under and cramp.

After an evaluation, I realized that Marilyn had many influences at work in her. Not only was she dealing with the symptoms of fibromyalgia, she was also confronted with what many call the "empty nest syndrome." But this woman did not seek pity. Instead, she sought the assistance of an excellent psychologist, who helped her learn some of the relaxation techniques described in chapter 6. She found music therapy and deep abdominal breathing especially helpful, particularly during stressful times.

Using a combination of treatment, including medication, exercise, moist heat, and the mind / body approach to healing, Marilyn was able to find relief. Choosing any one component of the treatment program alone will not give such outstanding relief. That is why I constantly encourage a total combination treatment program.

APPENDIX:
SUGGESTED EXERCISES
FOR FIBROMYALGIA PATIENTS

The following exercises are designed to build flexibility and strength in the neck, shoulders, and back. It is important to work toward a goal of doing these exercises twice a day, twenty repetitions each. At first you may only be able to do one to two repetitions of each exercise. That's a reasonable start. But as you gain strength and mobility, move into a twice daily, twenty repetitions each routine. If you have any pain or unusual feeling, stop the exercise and contact your physician.

Sometimes it is helpful to have some gentle assistance from a family member or friend. Your physician or physical therapist can show you how.

A word of caution: Do not hold your breath while performing any exercise. If you feel pain with any of the suggested exercises, stop the exercise and discuss it with your physician.

Neck Range-of-Motion Exercises

It is important to build strength in the neck as well as improve its mobility and flexibility. Because fibromyalgia causes stiffness and pain, these range-of-motion exercises will enable your body to perform more effectively. While flexion should be done while standing, the rest of the neck exercises can be performed sitting or standing, whichever is more comfortable for you.

FLEXION

While standing, look down and bend your chin forward to the chest. If you feel stiffness or pain, do not force the movement. Go as far as you can without straining yourself. If your muscle pain worsens with this or any exercise, stop until you have talked to your physician or physical therapist.

EXTENSION

Look up and bend your head back as far as possible without forcing any movement.

LATERAL FLEXION

Tilt your left ear to your left shoulder (but do not raise the shoulder). If you feel pain or resistance, do not force the motion.

Now tilt the ear to the right shoulder just as you did for the left ear (see figure 1).

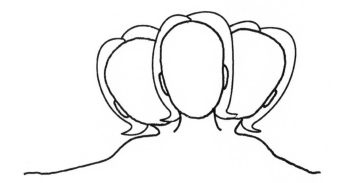

FIGURE 1. LATERAL FLEXION

ROTATION

Turn to look over your left shoulder. Try to make your chin even with your shoulder. Go as far as is comfortable, but do not force the movement.

Now turn and look over your right shoulder, as with the left.

Neck Isometric Exercises

Neck isometric exercises are more advanced exercises to help strengthen the muscles of the neck, which is most important in fibromyalgia. Try these gently and gradually after range of motion of your neck is improved as much as possible. Again, do not hold your breath.

ISOMETRIC FLEXION

1. Place hand on forehead. Try to look down while resisting the motion with your hand. Hold for six seconds, counting out loud.

2. Place your hands on the back of your head. Try to look up and back while resisting the motion with your hands. Hold for six seconds, counting out loud.

ISOMETRIC LATERAL FLEXION

Start with your head straight. Place your left hand just above your left ear (see figure 2 on page 171). Try to tilt your head to the left but resist the motion with your left hand. Hold for six seconds, counting out loud.

Now place your right hand just above your right ear. Try to tilt your head to the right but resist the movement with your right hand. Hold for six seconds, counting out loud.

ISOMETRIC ROTATION

Place your left hand above your ear and near your left forehead. Now try to look over your left shoulder, but resist the

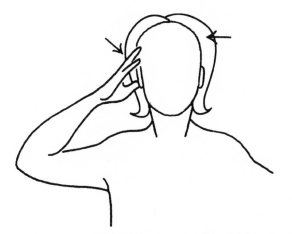

FIGURE 2. ISOMETRIC LATERAL FLEXION

motion with your left hand. The hand should not be placed on the jaw. Hold for six seconds, counting out loud.

Now place your right hand above your ear and near your right forehead. Try to look over your right shoulder but resist the motion with your right hand. Hold for six seconds, counting out loud.

Shoulder Range-of-Motion Exercises

The following five range-of-motion exercises will increase the flexibility of the shoulders and arms. Increasing the number of exercises will increase the strength of the arms.

SHOULDER EXTERNAL ROTATION

This exercise increases the motion you use to comb your hair. You may sit, stand, or lie down to do these exercises.

Clasp your hands behind your head. Pull your elbows together until they are as close as possible in front of your chin. Separate the elbows to the side as much as possible.

Repeat this, gradually increasing to five, then ten, then up to twenty repetitions. You may repeat these two or three times daily.

SHOULDER INTERNAL ROTATION

Shoulder internal rotation increases the flexibility of the shoulders. Using the same motions women use to fasten a bra in the back or men use to put a wallet in a back pocket, move your arms behind your back, as shown in figure 3 (see page 173). This exercise is best done standing and is often done in the shower using a washcloth to wash your upper back and a towel to dry it.

Put your hand behind your back, then put the other hand behind your back and cross the wrist as shown in the picture. Return the hands to rest at your side.

Repeat this twice daily, gradually increasing to five, then ten, then up to twenty repetitions per session.

SHOULDER FLEXION

Shoulder flexion holds both arms down at your sides. Raise the left arm straight up and reach overhead toward the ceiling. Now do the same with the right arm. Continue this motion as you alternate left-right-left-right.

Repeat twice daily, gradually increasing to five, then ten, then up to twenty repetitions per session.

SHOULDER ABDUCTION

Raise both arms straight out away from your sides, then raise each arm overhead toward the ceiling and up above your head. It doesn't matter whether you do this palm-up or palm-down.

If it's painful to do this exercise while sitting or standing, you can also do it lying on your bed, using a stick (a broom handle will do). As you raise your arms, hold the stick with

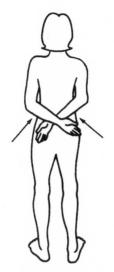

FIGURE 3. SHOULDER INTERNAL ROTATION

both hands and keep your arms straight, up over your head as far as possible. The strength of the less painful arm will help the painful arm move more easily.

Repeat this exercise, gradually increasing to five, then ten, then twenty repetitions, two or three times a day.

Once you have mastered the exercise, go to part two of this exercise, which involves raising your arm out to your side, one at a time, then making big circles slowly.

Repeat this exercise, gradually increasing to five, then ten, then twenty repetitions, two or three times a day.

SHOULDER GIRDLE ROTATION

This exercise can be done in a sitting or standing position and is fun to do during the day to relieve neck and shoulder tension and maintain shoulder girdle flexibility.

Roll shoulders in a forward circle, and raise shoulders toward the ears in a shrugging motion. Then, roll shoulders

back and your chest out, as in a military stance. Lower the
shoulders and bring them forward. Think of it as a simple
shoulder roll in a circle. Now reverse the process, rolling
your shoulder girdle in a backward circle.

Repeat this exercise, gradually increasing to five, then ten,
then twenty repetitions two or three times a day, if possible.

Back Exercises

As you do the following strengthening exercises, it is very
important that you breathe properly while holding a position.
Counting to six out loud will enable you to do this easily. If
you experience shortness of breath, stop and talk to your doctor or physical therapist.

CHEEK TO CHEEK
This is a convenient exercise because you can do it anywhere,
anytime, and practically in any position. It strengthens the
muscles of the buttocks that help support the back and the
legs. When sitting, you will actually raise up out of the chair
because of the contraction of the muscle groups in the buttocks.

Press your buttocks together and hold for a six-second
count. Relax and repeat. Gradually increase up to five, then
ten, then twenty repetitions.

PELVIC TILT
This is one of the best exercises you can do to strengthen your
abdominal muscles which in turn help support your back. It
will also help tone your stomach muscles. Do this exercise
lying on your back in bed or on the floor, whichever is more
comfortable.

Relax and raise your arms above your head. Keep your
knees bent. Now comes the tricky part! Tighten the muscles

of your lower abdomen and your buttocks at the same time to flatten your back against the floor or bed. Hold the flat back position for a six-second count. Now relax and repeat.

Repeat this exercise two or three times to start and work gradually to five, then ten, then twenty repetitions twice a day.

If you have trouble, contact your physical therapist or physician and have him or her demonstrate the exercise.

BRIDGING

This exercise strengthens the muscles in the back.

Lie on your back on the floor or in bed and bend your knees. Now lift your hips and buttocks off the bed or floor four to six inches, forcing the small of the back out flat; and tighten the buttock and hip muscles to maintain this position (see figure 4 below). Hold this position for a count of six seconds. Relax and lower your hips and buttocks to the floor or bed.

Repeat this exercise, gradually increasing up to five, then ten, then twenty repetitions as tolerated. Repeat twice daily, if possible.

PARTIAL SIT-UP

This is one of the more vigorous exercises. Its purpose is to build abdominal strength, which will give the back greater support. To do this exercise, lie on your bed or on the floor,

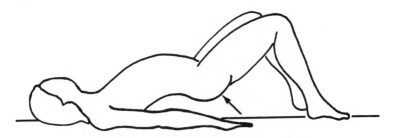

FIGURE 4. A BRIDGING EXERCISE

whichever is more comfortable. Lie on your back with your knees bent. Raise your head and shoulder blades off the floor or bed (see figure 5 below). Hold that position for a six-second count. Slowly return to the beginning position. Repeat.

Start this exercise slowly, with one or two repetitions, until your body adjusts. Gradually increase to five, then ten repetitions.

BACK EXTENSION

For this exercise to strengthen the back muscles, lie on your bed or on the floor in a prone (stomach-down) position. A pillow may be used under the stomach to help make this position more comfortable.

Raise your head, arms, and legs off the floor. Do not bend your knees. This must be done with your body straight in extension. Hold for six seconds while you count out loud. Relax and repeat.

Gradually increase up to five, then ten repetitions. If you experience discomfort, check with your physician or physical therapist before you continue.

CAT-CAMEL

Do not do this exercise for strengthening the back muscles if you have very painful knees, ankles, or hands, as it places pressure on these areas.

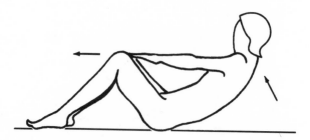

FIGURE 5. A PARTIAL SIT-UP EXERCISE

The position for this exercise is a crawling position (see figure 6 below). Hands must be directly under your shoulders. Take a deep breath and arch your back as a frightened cat does, lowering your head. Hold that position for six seconds, counting out loud. Now exhale and drop the arched back slowly, raising your head.

Start this exercise slowly with one or two repetitions. Increase up to five and then ten repetitions, if possible.

WALL PUSH

This exercise is good for the back because it encourages the body extension positions.

Stand spread-eagle, with your hands against a wall. Now arch your back inward slowly.

Gradually increase repetitions from one to five or more. This exercise is fun because you can do it anytime you feel you need a good body stretch. Repeat two times daily.

BACK FLEXIBILITY

Lie on your back on the floor with knees bent and feet flat on the floor. Raise hands toward the ceiling. Now move arms and head to the right, while the knees move to the left. Reverse

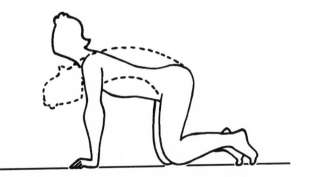

FIGURE 6. A CAT-CAMEL EXERCISE

the above, then repeat. Gradually increase up to five and then ten repetitions twice daily.

BICYCLING

Lying on your back, move your feet and legs in the air as if you were riding a bicycle. Count to six and relax. Repeat, then gradually increase to five and then ten repetitions once or twice daily, if tolerated.

REFERENCES AND SUPPORTING RESEARCH

"Alternative Medicine: The Facts." *Consumer Reports* (January 1994): 51.

Antonelli, Mary Ann, M.D., and Robert L. Vawter, M.D. "Nonarticular Pain Syndromes." *Nonarticular Disorders* 91 (February 1992): 95–104.

Arthritis Foundation. *Fibromyalgia (Fibrositis),* 1992.

Benson, Herbert, M.D., and Eileen M. Stuart, R.N., M.S. *The Wellness Book.* New York: Birch Lane Press, 1992.

"Bluer Than Blue." *Involved* (Fall 1993): 2.

Croft, Peter, Joanna Schollum, and Alan Silman. "Population Study of Tender Point Counts and Pain as Evidence of Fibromyalgia." *British Medical Journal* 309 (September 1994): 696(4).

Dranov, Paula. "Am I Sick or Am I Tired?" *Ladies Home Journal* 106 (September 1989): 120(4).

Duna, George F., M.D., and William S. Wilke, M.D. "Diagnosis, Etiology and Therapy of Fibromyalgia." *Comprehensive Therapy* 1993; 19(2): 60–63.

"Emotions: How They Affect Your Body." *Discover* (November 1984): 35.

"Exercise: A Little Helps a Lot." *Consumer Reports on Health* (August 1994): 89.

Ferguson, Pamela. *The Self-Shiatsu Handbook.* New York: Perigee Books, 1995.

Ferraccioli George, et al. "EMG-Biofeedback Training in Fibromyalgia Syndrome." *Journal of Rheumatology* 14 (1987): 820–25.

"Fibromyalgia Unrelenting." *The Back Letter* 9 (May 1994): 60–61.

Geel, Stanley E. "The Fibromyalgia Syndrome: Musculoskeletal Pathophysiology." *Seminars in Arthritis and Rheumatism* 23 (April 1994): 347–53.

Griffin, Katherine. "A Whiff of Things to Come." *Health* 6 (November / December 1992): 34.

Hagen, Kathryn. "Feeling Better with Music." *Arthritis Today* 7 (March / April 1993): 19.

Hagglund, K. J., W. E. Deuser, S. P. Buckelew, J. Hewett, and D. R. Kay. "Weather, Beliefs About Weather, and Disease Severity Among Patients with Fibromyalgia." *Arthritis Care Res.* (September 1994): 130–35.

Kjeldsen-Kragh, J., M. Haugen, C. F. Borchgrevink, and O. Forre. "Vegetarian Diet for Patients with Rheumatoid Arthritis." *Clinical Rheumatology* (December 1994): 649.

Kline, Nathan S. *From Sad to Glad.* New York: Ballantine Books, 1974.

Leventhal, L. J., E. G. Boyce, and R. B. Zuerier. "Treatment of Rheumatoid Arthritis with Blackcurrant Seed Oil. *British Journal of Rheumatology* 33 (September 1994): 847–52.

Locke, Andrew, M.D., and Nicola Gedees, M.D. *The Woman's Guide to Homeopathy.* New York: St. Martin's Press, 1994.

Lorenzen, I. "Fibromyalgia: A Clinical Challenge." *Journal of Internal Medicine* (1994): 199–203.

McClaflin, Richard R., M.D. "Myofascial Pain Syndrome." *Myofascial Pain Syndrome* 96 (August 1994): 56–73.

McIlwain, Harris, M.D., Debra Fulghum Bruce, Joel Silverfield, M.D., Michael Burnette, M.D., and Bernard Germaine, M.D. *Winning with Back Pain.* New York: John Wiley, 1994.

———. *Winning with Chronic Pain.* New York: Prometheus Books, 1994.

Nathan, Ronald G., Thomas E. Staats, and Paul J. Rosch. *The Doctor's Guide to Instant Stress Relief.* New York: G. P. Putnam, 1987.

Novakoski, Frank, A.T.C. "The Benefits of Weight Training." *Living Well Today* (January 1994): 6.

Nye, David A. "Fibromyalgia: A Guide for Patients." http://www.hsc.missour . . . yalgia/docs/fm-md.html. 1995.

"Optimistic Prognosis for Fibromyalgia Sufferers: Work Disability Uncommon in Decade-Long Study." *The Back Letter* 9 (December 1994): 133(3).

Pillemer, Stanley R., M.D. *The Fibromyalgia Syndrome.* New York: Haworth Press, 1994.

"Probing the Mystery of Fibromyalgia." *Health News* 12 (October 1994): 1.

Selye, H. *Stress Without Distress.* New York: New American Library, 1975.

Sorvino, A. Ronald; Kalstrom, Elizabeth; Abel, Gene G. "Biofeedback for Musculoskeletal Pain." *Journal of the American Medical Association.* December 8, 1993, Vol. 270, n. 22, pp. 2736(1).

Wartik, Nancy. "Making Sense of Aromatherapy." *American Health* (October 1995): 73–74.

White, Kevin P., Manfred Harth, and Robert W. Teasell. "Work Disability Evaluation and the Fibromyalgia Syndrome." *Seminars in Arthritis and Rheumatism* 24 (June 1995): 371(10).

Wilke, William S. "Treatment of Resistant Fibromyalgia." *Rheumatic Disease Clinics of North America* (February 1995): 247–60.

Wolfe, Frederick, M.D. "When to Diagnose Fibromyalgia." *Rheumatic Disease Clinics of North America.* 20, no. 2 (May 1994): 485–99.

Wurtman, Judith J. "Depression and Weight Gain: The Serotonin Connection." *Journal of Affective Disorders* 29 (1993): 183–92.

Yunus, Muhammad B., M.D. "Fibromyalgia Syndrome: A Need for Uniform Classification." *Journal of Rheumatology* 10 (1983): 841–44.

INDEX